Childbirth in a Technocratic Age

Childbirth in a Technocratic Age

The Documentation of Women's Expectations and Experiences

Elizabeth Soliday

CAMBRIA PRESS

Amherst, New York

Requests for permission should be directed to:
permissions@cambriapress.com, or mailed to:
Cambria Press
20 Northpointe Parkway, Suite 188
Amherst, NY 14228

Library of Congress Cataloging-in-Publication Data

Soliday, Elizabeth.
Childbirth in a technocratic age : the documentation of women's expectations and experiences / Elizabeth Soliday.
p. cm.
Includes bibliographical references and index.
ISBN 978-1-60497-798-1 (alk. paper)
1. Childbirth—Psychological aspects. 2. Mother and child. I. Title.

RG652.S58 2012
618.4—dc23

2012003356

To mothers everywhere, and to LHH and VCH

Table of Contents

List of Figure and Table

Preface

Childbirth is more admirable than conquest, more amazing than self-defense, and as courageous as either one.

—Gloria Steinem

I recently watched a television sitcom that unfolded in the following way: Giving birth for the first time, the lead character labors without incident at work, supported by other women, before her husband whisks her away to the hospital in a limousine. Another man, a physician she has never met, enters the hospital room, announces that he is in charge, and refuses her request to see her regular female obstetrician. The lead character labors miserably in her hospital bed awhile before her husband convinces her—against her wishes to go medication free—to accept an epidural; the audience then sees the lead in anesthetically induced bliss. When the physician reenters the scene, the lead pushes as ordered, but to no avail: The physician proclaims that the baby's head is "too big" and that cesarean delivery is "not a choice," and he leaves to prepare for surgery. The lead's husband assures her that surgery is necessary because the doctor said so. In the final scene, the lead sits comfortably in her hospital bed, any grief over having missed the birth experience she had expected seemingly washed away by the perfect baby she holds in her arms.

I cannot know whether the writers of that sitcom intended it, but the program captured what 21st-century U.S. women have come to expect as normal and acceptable in childbirth. First, hospital birth managed by experts (as opposed to mothers) is viewed as superior to any alternative, whatever that may be. Labor without an epidural is agonizing and, more important, unnecessary. Labor with an epidural is pleasant. Fetal heads are large, the birth canal is narrow, and cesarean surgery is an excellent—if not the only—solution. Obstetric medical procedures produce perfect babies with no negative consequences. Mothers' voices do not matter because men—husbands, doctors, limousine drivers—are in charge.

Those favoring this prevailing hospital-based, doctor-centered maternal-care paradigm argue that it offers mothers and babies greater safety than any alternative. It is also tirelessly argued that increasingly aggressive obstetric intervention like that shown in the sitcom has come in response to worries over litigation; birthing women and juries view active intervention as more responsible than allowing nature to take its course. Both points are certainly debatable, as this text's scientific data and maternal reports make clear. Less debatable, however, is that the prevailing maternal-care paradigm generates big income for large, powerful institutions and associated practitioners, especially when childbirth proceeds quickly and involves multiple interventions, such as epidurals and cesareans.

But like the lead character in the sitcom just described, some mothers want to experience childbirth according to nature's and their own bodies' design. Also like the lead character in the sitcom, most are forced to do so in traditional institutions because they have few practical alternatives and because, like most American women, they are subject to cultural assumptions and related efforts by major medical organizations to promote the idea that anything except institutional birth is dangerous and irresponsible. Granted, medical institutions have worked to make hospital birth more appealing; efforts include dressing up maternity suites, offering tasty meals, and stocking rooms with consumer goodies like iPod docking stations and video cameras. However, as the sitcom made so plain, the fancy dressing cannot disguise the fact that for the most part, the power structure created by men drives treatment decisions and technological intrusion into the decidedly female-owned childbirth domain, eventually convincing women that they want or must have it that way.

I believe that this "high-tech, low-touch" model of maternal care persists because technology is being used to replace the caring and comfort historically provided by birthing mothers' families and communities, and because those more human supports are fast disappearing in contemporary U.S. life. Whether for these or for other reasons, this care model prevails, and available statistics on its intensification—for example, the cesarean delivery rate increased by nearly 1% over the course of my preparing this book—point to a most logical yet preposterous conclusion. That is, technology and those who operate it will completely replace the limited role that most mothers (and sitcom actresses) have in childbirth today. All deliveries will be scheduled and will occur by cesarean. Women will no longer feel labor contractions except when they unexpectedly begin before the date set for surgery. Technicians, rather than mothers, will then take full ownership of the kind of triumph that many birthing mothers in this book described. In other words, the contemporary culture at large seems determined to overwrite nature's most marvelous design, the ability to birth another body from one's own. The culture at large seems similarly determined to discourage women from taking full advantage of the power their bodies and minds possess in childbirth and of the established health benefits for both mothers and newborns of supported childbirth with minimal intervention.

Without question, early 21st-century maternal care is approaching a crisis state requiring one to stop and reflect on the present situation, which directions it might take, and why. Adrienne Rich in her 1976 classic *Of Woman Born* wrote that medical professionals, usually men, have written more about childbirth than any other group has, and that "the one group whose opinions and documentation we long to have—the mothers—are, as usual, almost entirely unheard-from" (p. 130). In the absence of documented maternal accounts of childbirth, those on the outside can only guess at what really happened in childbirth at any place or time, whether among a Polynesian tribe 1,000 years ago or in a North American hospital two days ago. I wrote this book on women's reported childbirth expectations and experiences for the millions of women who, like the sitcom character, have endured childbirth with their voices unheard; I hope to alert readers to the critical need to treat birthing women of all persuasions decently and humanely.

Like all good stories, the mothers' pregnancy-to-postpartum accounts contained in this volume make apparent the tremendous physical and psychic transformations of childbirth, along with its attendant joy, vigor, misery, and rage. Like the stories of women generations before that went unrecognized and unrecorded, my interviewees' accounts contribute to the eternal tale of how humans come to be. Alongside the scientific information in this text, these mothers' stories illustrate how society views motherhood more generally in this cultural time and space. In the name of continuing to better the lives of mothers, their offspring, and those who care for them, I hope this account inspires readers, whether they are mothers or not, to appreciate and celebrate the mothers in their lives and around the globe.

Acknowledgments

The author wishes to thank the mothers who generously shared their childbirth accounts, as well as Randi Hutter Epstein, Redmond Reams, the WSU Vancouver College of Liberal Arts and Office of Research, the Cambria Press editors and staff, and the anonymous reviewers.

Childbirth in a Technocratic Age

Chapter 1

Maternal Expectations in 21st-Century U.S. Birth Culture

I'm not worried at all ... I'm going in there carefree, knowing things are optimal.

—Maggie, second-time mother, on her upcoming hospital birth with an expected epidural

Like so many of the nearly four million women who give birth in the United States each year, my interviewee Maggie (a pseudonym) anticipated a worry-free vaginal delivery made safer by traditional hospital care and made easier with an advanced pain treatment available only in that setting. For a handful of women, the various forces influencing their ultimate childbirth experiences—personal and institutional resources, professional practices and routines, and somewhere in the mix, their own desires—come together in an almost magical way to produce an outcome not too far from what they had imagined. But for many more, Maggie included, those same forces collide in unanticipated ways, producing an unwelcome mismatch between childbirth expectations and subsequent experiences that stand to create unsettling, powerful, and lasting impressions of this otherwise life-affirming event.

The cause of mismatches between maternal expectations and experiences is not, I would argue, a simple matter of how any one woman's body behaves in childbirth, though one most certainly cannot dismiss that factor. Instead, today's women are living in a culture characterized by conflicting forces that play out in labor and delivery. On the one hand, contemporary mothers have available to them grand opportunities that were unavailable to previous generations, such as ready and unrestricted access to information on childbirth and obstetric care (e.g., Murkoff & Mazel, 2008; Simkin, Bolding, Keppler, & Durham, 2010), hard-won rights to participate in maternal treatment decisions (e.g., American College of Obstetricians and Gynecologists [ACOG], 2008; Anonymous, 1977), and dozens of childbirth options designed to improve childbirth's safety and quality. Constraining those opportunities, however, are gross inequities in health-care resources, with obstetric practice dictated as much by resource availability, institutional policy, physician convenience, and legal concerns as by maternal interests and needs (e.g., Armstrong, 2000; Block, 2008).

Take, for example, baths during labor: nearly half of women who labor in tubs find that baths provide effective pain relief (Declercq, Sakala, & Corry, 2002), but because of costs, professional resistance to changing traditional practitioner-centered treatment, and institutional concerns about risks that do not exist, access to this option is hardly widespread. One of the mothers in my study living in a large southeastern city reported that "only one hospital, one practitioner" offered ready access to a tub for laboring, and securing that practitioner's care required the mother to change insurance plans. Another of my study mothers labored several hours in water but was instructed to leave the tub to facilitate placement of an internal fetal monitor—involving an electrode inserted through the mother's vagina and placed in a tiny surgical cut in the baby's scalp—for reasons she did not understand. Two other study mothers mentioned wanting birthing tubs but wondered whether the hospitals to which their public insurance restricted them would allow their use.

Additionally, the developmental status of obstetric interventions used with increasing frequency, such as labor induction and planned surgical delivery, constrains their potential to consistently deliver promised benefits with predictable or known consequences. As becomes evident in later chapters, only a few women who had full faith in medical and pharmacological treatments as the key to worry-free birth described their subsequent experiences in positive terms. A few mothers said their epidural relieved pain as anticipated; a few women had generally positive experiences with planned cesarean surgery. But many more found themselves surprised by the failure of an anticipated treatment to fulfill their expectations.

This brings us back to Maggie, whose decision to plan an epidural led her to feel "carefree" about her upcoming birth. When she went into labor a few months later, she traveled to the hospital in the early morning hours, and because there was a long line of patients awaiting help from the single available anesthesiologist, Maggie waited her turn. The anesthesiologist finally arrived and successfully placed Maggie's epidural—a procedure involving careful insertion of several needles and a catheter in the lower spine—after several painful attempts. Unfortunately, like a small but significant percentage of women, Maggie found the epidural "totally ineffective," adding, "I could feel everything, every contraction, the tearing. And the stitching up." Afterwards, Maggie's nurse reportedly told her she had been "lucky" that she had not contracted a "flesh-eating staph infection" from the procedure, as the mother next door had, leading Maggie to say she wished she'd "never gotten the thing" because "it didn't work anyway."

In the context of the contemporary childbirth culture, I asked what early 21st-century mothers expected to happen in childbirth, how their experiences matched their expectations, and how satisfied they were with the process overall. Childbirth involves a mother's physical self, her psyche, her social role, and her community at large, and that depth of involvement alone sufficiently justifies any examination of maternal experiences. From a psychological perspective, however, better understanding the match between expected and lived childbirth experiences is critical because mismatches between the two can result in increased postpartum maternal distress (e.g., Ayers & Pickering, 2005; Crowe & von Baeyer, 1989); early postpartum distress can, in turn, result in more difficult mother–newborn interactions and longer term relationship difficulties (Cicchetti, Rogosch, & Toth, 1998; van Doesum, Riksen-Walraven, Hosman, & Hoefnagels, 2008).

On a broader scale, amplifying the maternal voice is essential in addressing a pervasive and powerful contemporary cultural childbirth message that a healthy newborn's arrival should erase any maternal misgivings about whatever toll labor and delivery take, a notion perfectly reflected in one mother's words, "Hello—your baby's healthy! We're all shooting for the end product here. So what if you didn't push it out and got a c-section?" Sadly, the "end product," no matter how healthy or perfect, cannot undo what came before, and childbirth memories, good and bad, last for years (Simkin, 1992; Waldenstrom, 2003) and influence subsequent childbearing plans and experiences (Gottvall & Waldenstrom, 2002; Hildingsson, Radestad, Rubertsoon, & Waldenstrom, 2002; Pang, Leung, Lan, & Hang Chung, 2008). Evidencing the persistence of childbirth memories, another study mother, whose baby arrived healthy, said of her planned cesarean delivery followed by abysmal postoperative care: "If this had been my first experience … I would have been like, 'Oh my gosh, don't ever let me have any more kids' if this is what it means." Giving voice to how mothers' experiences of childbirth may align with or stray from expectations acknowledges their perspectives as worthy, valid, and as central to ongoing discourse surrounding maternal needs and quality care.

FEATURES OF CONTEMPORARY U.S. BIRTH CULTURE INFLUENCING MATERNAL EXPECTATIONS

Over 99% of 21st-century U.S. women deliver their newborns in traditional hospitals (Martin et al., 2010). Physicians, whose training generally focuses on treating things that go wrong rather than things that go right, attended 93% of hospital births as of 2007 (Martin et al., 2010). Midwives attended most of the remaining hospital deliveries, and though they are trained to view childbirth as a normal, healthy process, they are still subject to hospital protocol, which currently translates into rates for common obstetric procedure use of over 50%. This means any hospital-birthing mother has a better than one in two chance of receiving *some* procedure in a hospital birth—adding up to over two million U.S. women a year who receive hospital obstetric intervention whether they had planned on it or not. With contemporary birth interventions occurring at these rates, mothers who achieve birth experiences consistent with their earlier views, particularly those pursuing intervention-free birth, constitute a true statistical minority.

One of the greatest contributors to current intervention rates is the emphasis on controlling the process, most often by reducing the time women spend in pregnancy, labor, and delivery with medical procedures to manage when labor begins (onset), its duration, and the newborn's arrival. As but one indication of the contemporary "race to the finish" childbirth orientation, for first-time mothers, U.S. hospital protocols commonly set 12 hours as a safe limit for "normal" first-stage labor (Zhang et al., 2010), whereas the World Health Organization (WHO) grants women 20 hours in a first birth (2006a). To move labor along, labor-acceleration procedures are frequently introduced. For example, in mothers who plan to deliver vaginally, labor typically starts on its own (spontaneously) sometime between the 38th and 41st week of pregnancy, but decreasing numbers of women wait for natural labor because of the growing use of an artificial, hospital-based procedure known as medical labor induction. In 1980, only 1.1% of mothers underwent labor induction (DeFrances, Cullen, & Kozak, 2007); in the early 21st century, hospital records and maternal reports yielded figures ranging from 23–41% (Declercq, Sakala, Corry, & Appelbaum, 2006). (More on labor induction and related controversies appears in chapters 2 and 3).

Additional statistics show how pervasive other labor-acceleration strategies have become. One of the simplest, nearly universal, but often unanticipated strategies is intravenous (IV) fluid administration: Doubling the most commonly administered IV fluid dosage may reduce first-stage labor by up to two hours[1] (O'Sullivan & Scrutton, 2003). Amniotomy, or inserting a crochet hook–like instrument through the mother's vagina and cervix to rupture the bag of waters surrounding the fetus, is practiced on the premise that it can kick-start or speed up labor (Vincent, 2005). In 1980, only about 3.2% of women reportedly underwent amniotomy (DeFrances et al., 2007); by 2006, the rate had shot up to 59% (Declercq et al., 2006). Intravenous infusion of the drug oxytocin, commonly known by the brand name Pitocin, induces and accelerates labor by increasing uterine contractions. Oxytocin administration saw a threefold jump from 17.4% of mothers in 1997 to 55% in 2006 (Declercq et al., 2006; Ventura, Martin, Curtin, & Mathews, 1999). Rates of other procedures, including episiotomy (surgical cutting of the vaginal opening to facilitate newborn exit) and forceps or vacuum assistance, have actually decreased, offset by increased cesarean delivery (Martin et al., 2010).

Two other obstetric procedures used with vaginally delivering mothers warrant mention because they have come to be used routinely and figure into hospital labor and delivery time lines. Epidural labor analgesia (discussed in more detail in chapters 4 and 5), involving an opiate drug injection into the spinal column during labor (and therefore sometimes labeled *spinal labor analgesia*), slows uterine contractions. Epidural rates have increased threefold since 1981 and are now used in 71–78% of all birthing mothers (Declercq et al., 2006; Deering, Zaret, McGaha, & Satin, 2007; Hawkins, Gibbs, Orleans, Martin-Salvaj, & Beaty, 1997). Intrapartum antibiotic prophylaxis (IAP) is an IV drug infusion administered in labor to prevent maternal-to-fetal transmission of a common adult infection, group B streptococcus (GBS). In 2002, the U.S. Centers for Disease Control and Prevention (CDC) called for testing all mothers for GBS in their final weeks of pregnancy in order to plan for IAP. Despite controversy surrounding IAP's risks and its ineffectiveness in reducing GBS-related newborn deaths (Baltimore, 2007; Ohlsson & Shah, 2009; Stoll et al., 2002), up to 30% of contemporary U.S. mothers receive IAP (CDC, 2002).

An additional consideration is that labor induction, labor acceleration, epidurals, and IAP are infrequently delivered in isolation because one intervention often leads to another (Simpson, & Thorman, 2005); this is referred to as the "cascade of interventions" and translates into multiple points of potential deviation from childbirth expectations. For example, labor contractions in a mother whose labor was induced might not become regular, in which case oxytocin might be increased as her deadline for delivery nears. With contractions of increased intensity, the mother might request an epidural, which would slow her labor, increasing the need for more oxytocin, and so on. This use of one procedure to address the shortcomings of another led some of my study mothers to describe their labor experiences "like a rollercoaster" or as involving "being hooked up to all kinds of tubes and wires."

Perhaps the most dramatic deviation from an expected "normal," vaginal birth is cesarean delivery. Of the approximate 32% early 21st-century cesarean deliveries (Martin et al., 2010; Meikle, Steiner, Zhang, & Lawrence, 2005; United States National Institutes of Health, 2006), about half are the so-called labored or emergency cesareans performed on women who had been in labor when someone determined that it was time to terminate labor with surgery in the interest of maternal or fetal health. Labored cesareans should be distinguished from the remaining half of cesarean surgeries that are planned—that is, scheduled months or weeks ahead of time to occur around the baby's due date, allowing mothers to forego labor entirely. For both labored and planned cesareans, uniform guidelines on appropriate medical cause are vague or nonexistent; this and related issues are discussed in chapters 6 and 7.

Both within the medical community and among the public at large, routine practice of procedures such as labor induction, IAP, and cesarean surgery is frequently supported with the argument that such procedures make childbirth safer overall, and that though the procedures carry their own risks, they are preferable to what *could happen* if the interventions were not used. Consequently, the argument continues, how could a responsible mother trade the known risks of a perhaps unnecessary birth procedure for the unknown risks of proceeding without it, even if this means violating her childbirth expectations? Furthermore, how could a mother reasonably claim any misgivings about expectations gone awry as long as her baby, the "end product," arrived in good condition?

According to available statistics, more intervention does not seem to have kept mothers and newborns any safer: Maternal health has remained unchanged alongside increased procedures over the past three to four decades, with fewer than 1,000 U.S. mothers dying in childbirth per year[2] (Hoyert, 2007) since the 1970s. Severe childbirth-related morbidities (complications) such as hemorrhage, serious infection, blood clots, and uterine rupture have remained constant since 1998, occurring in 3–6% of annual births, or over 100,000 women (Clark et al., 2008; Kuklina et al., 2009). And neonatal health—infant mortality, preterm birth, and low birth weight—has *worsened* slightly over the past several decades alongside increased obstetric intervention (MacDorman, & Mathews, 2008; United States Centers for Disease Control and Prevention & Health Resources and Services Administration, 2009), particularly cesarean delivery (see chapter 5). Moreover, evidence of climbing obstetric intervention rates among young healthy and less healthy mothers alike contradicts any argument that more intervention is necessary to treat an increasingly obese or older maternal population.

At the time of their development, most aggressive obstetric interventions (e.g., labor acceleration and cesarean delivery) were designed to treat mothers and newborns at high risk of imminent peril. More recently, however, those same interventions have been downgraded for use in otherwise healthy, normal, low-risk cases. For example, labor induction was once reserved for the minute percentage of mothers whose pregnancies had exceeded 41 weeks, but the procedure has been extended to patients in whom only minor or even no complications exist, such as mothers whose amniotic fluid is judged low or who simply wish to bring the pregnancy to an end. In other words, increased intervention has not translated into any striking benefits in terms of maternal or newborn safety because those on the receiving end were just as safe or safer before the intervention.

Nevertheless, any mother who during the course of childbirth hears that she or her offspring faces some risk could easily lose sight of statistics as she deals with her immediate situation, no matter how mild or serious. Mothers in this study reported hearing providers speak of the dangers of carrying the baby beyond the due date, such as more difficult childbirth or an aging placenta or the risk of "stressing their babies out" by continuing to labor. Under the stress of labor and hearing unsettling news from a trusted birth attendant, a mother may understandably prefer to accept the known risk of a potentially unnecessary procedure rather than face the unknown risk of what could happen if she chose to forgo it—even if the intervention derailed her expected experience.

However, the known risks of often casually used contemporary birth interventions are far from minimal. For example, as I discuss more fully in chapter 2, labor induction carries increased risk of infections, blood loss, and hemorrhage (Caughey et al., 2009; Dublin, Lyndon-Rochelle, Kaplan, Watts, & Critchlow, 2000; Mozurkewich, Chilimigras, Koepke, Keeton, & King, 2009). As another example, IAP has been associated with increased maternal and neonatal yeast infections, and up to 20% of children of IAP-treated mothers may later develop resistance to certain antibiotics (Baltimore, 2007; Ohlsson & Shah, 2009; Stoll et al., 2002). Furthermore, treating more women with IAP may trigger growth of antibiotic resistant bacteria, particularly *E. coli* (Baltimore et al., 2007). The lack of systematic studies on the intervention cascade—labor induction, amniotomy, epidural, and oxytocin—reminds one that more is currently unknown than known about how combined interventions affect short- and long-term maternal health.

As has been the case over the past century in the United States, mothers today generally place their faith in their birth attendants, believing it wisest to trust obstetric professionals and the knowledge they have gained through formal training as opposed to relying on their own maternal instinct or wisdom. Similarly, mothers generally assume that their birth attendants recommend particular obstetric interventions because the occasion warrants it. However, in the United States' privately financed health-care system, obstetric institutions and many of their associated birth attendants are forced to attend to the economic bottom line, which may mean using interventions to move more patients more quickly through labor and delivery. Contemporary medicine has also shifted its orientation from one of treating serious illness in its latter stages to intervening earlier, when the risk or signs of illness first arise. But pregnancy, labor, and delivery are not medical problems; they are normal physical processes that occur without complications in the vast majority of well-nourished women.

Certainly, I am not the first to note that contemporary obstetric treatment parallels aspects of early to mid-20th-century obstetric practice—particularly in the inappropriate use of interventions that lack sound scientific support. In the 1950s, obstetric nurses routinely positioned actively laboring mothers on their backs, strapping their hands, chests, and sometimes even legs to the labor bed to "prevent contamination of the sterile field" (Schultz, 1958, p. 152) before knocking them out with general anesthesia to erase memories of labor and delivery (Epstein, 2010). Might readers 50 years from now view early 21st-century rates of contemporary procedures like labor induction as similarly inhumane?

One bright spot in this otherwise gloomy picture of contemporary obstetric care is that today's mothers have ethical and legal protections that arose partly from mid-20th-century treatment, including the right to access information on all obstetric medical procedures and nonmedical alternatives and the right to collaborate in decision making (e.g., ACOG, 2008; American Medical Association, 1990; Anonymous, 1977). Along with those rights, of course, come responsibilities, such as reviewing treatment information, making decisions for oneself, and remaining healthy. Birthing mothers, however, are responsible not just for themselves but also for their offspring, putting them in a complex position when it comes to medical decision making. If mothers assert their rights in the course of their obstetric care, they may be subject to internal and external criticism and even legal action (e.g., Colb, 2004) because they exercise their autonomy instead of complying with medical authority. If they submit to medical authority, they may eventually question their own competence to make decisions or their ability to act responsibly on their offspring's behalf.

In sum, contemporary U.S. birth culture, including obstetric practices and the larger context in which those practices occur, places mothers at high risk of seeing their birth experiences diverge further from their birth expectations than in any other historical time or place. With maternal well-being central in the development and maintenance of strong, healthy mother–child relationships, it is essential to examine contemporary maternal expectations and their subsequent lived experiences of labor and delivery.

Previous Research on Expectations and Experiences

Research on matches between expectations and subsequent experiences emphasizes the centrality of one's subjective view as opposed to external or objective measures of how a given experience might have turned out. In contemporary childbirth culture, in which the view that the "end product" trumps whatever a mother might have had to endure and in which scientific indicators are valued more highly than experiential perspectives, attention to maternal subjective accounts becomes paramount. To put it more plainly, I take an example from one of my interviewees, a first-time mother who expressed persistent, negative thoughts about her birth experience that, contrary to her expectations of proceeding drug-free (her term), instead involved medical labor induction, an epidural, and ongoing oxytocin administration. From a contemporary obstetric perspective, the birth proceeded without complication and resulted in the delivery of a healthy newborn. Both perspectives might be valid, but the mother's view on her overall experience as widely divergent from what she had defined as normal would necessarily be the more critical driver of her later thoughts and feelings because she most directly experienced the events.

In psychological terms, an experience *confirms* an expectation when it meets it (expectancy confirmation); an experience *disconfirms* or *violates* an expectation when it deviates from it (expectancy violation).

In a most general sense, experiences deviating from earlier expectations symbolize randomness and unpredictability, and that sense, in turn, presumably leads to the negative emotions often tied to expectancy violations (Olson, Roese, & Zanna, 1996). As a process involving a woman's physical self as well as that of her fetus—not to mention her family and care providers and institutions—childbirth would seem, at least on the surface, to carry a particularly high likelihood of some unexpected occurrence. Not surprising, then, is the report that mothers' childbirth experiences generally violate their expectations (Gibbins & Thomson, 2001). Along similar lines, previous childbirth experience does not necessarily lead to better matched expectations and experiences (Booth & Meltzoff, 1984; Stolte, 1987), though primiparous (first-time) mothers may hold less realistic expectations of personal control over the childbirth process (Green, Coupland, & Kitzinger, 1998).

Poorly matched childbirth expectations and experiences are associated with negative maternal emotional consequences. For example, researchers Ayers and Pickering (2005) reported that poorly matched childbirth expectations and experiences corresponded to negative maternal views on the birth experience overall, which extended to more intense postpartum pain reported by mothers whose childbirth expectations were violated. Increasingly, a poor match between expectations and experiences involves the application of some unanticipated obstetric treatment, such as labor acceleration and episiotomy (treated in detail later in this chapter), which has been associated with lower maternal satisfaction with childbirth (Slade, MacPherson, Hume, & Maresh, 1993).

Some would argue that mothers have only limited influence or control over the degree to which their childbirth experiences match their expectations because birth is a complex physiological process involving multiple players. Yet according to Fiske and Taylor (1991), simply holding more or less positive expectations does seem to have some influence, and this effect has been demonstrated in birthing mothers. For example, among a large number of Belgian and Dutch mothers, those holding high expectations for good birth experiences in turn reported better childbirth experiences overall, and this held particularly true for those birthing at home

(Christiaens, Verhaeghe, & Bracke, 2008). Similarly, Green, Coupland, and Kitzinger (1990; 1998) reported that positive expectations related to a greater sense of control and a better birth experience, whereas negative expectations corresponded to more negative outcomes.

It may be that those who hold high expectations behave in ways to bring their experiences closer to what they ultimately anticipate (Miller & Turnbull, 1986). Among this study's mothers, for example, one who anticipated a medication-free hospital birth purchased a birth hypnosis home-study kit, made an audiotape of "birth affirmations" to use during labor and delivery, and requested that her wishes for natural birth written into her medical record. Dozens of mothers in this study seeking one approach to childbirth or another sought practitioners supportive of their interests in the hopes of achieving what they anticipated.

Overall, previous research has identified a connection between maternal expectations and experiences, and mismatches between the two have been associated with negative feelings toward the birth experience. Involved in the match between expectations and experiences may be the original quality of maternal expectations, obstetric intervention, and the birth setting; previous childbirth experience is less important. This research has limited relevance to contemporary U.S. mothers, however, because nearly all studies were conducted outside the United States, where health-care systems and cultural views differ; the unique context in which contemporary U.S. mothers are functioning, characterized by unprecedented options and constraints, will necessarily have some bearing on their expectations and on the extent to which their subsequent experiences match them.

Researcher Preconceptions and Biases

A critical step in the research process, particularly the approach I used in this study (described later in this chapter) is to identify one's preconceptions and biases and continually reflect on those over the course of the work (Moustakas, 1994). My research and clinical training prepared me to construct research materials, conduct interviews, and analyze data in ways that maximize objectivity. It is, however, only fair that I make plain certain of my biases related to this endeavor. My very choice to study pregnancy and childbirth shows a bias towards the topic itself, one that I have maintained since I enrolled in my first undergraduate psychology course.

Because of that interest, I sought graduate and postgraduate clinical training in major urban medical-center obstetrics and gynecology, neonatology, and pediatrics units. I did consultation-liaison work—that is, physicians requested my psychological assessments or intervention services when needed. In obstetrics, my cases included, for example, mothers with little or no social support, women whose psychological status raised questions about their safety or their ability to parent, and mothers grieving fetal or neonatal death. From those experiences, I learned firsthand about the enormous institutional pressures under which obstetric caregivers work. I also learned that on occasion, mothers present needs that no institution or professional could meet. In contrast, I witnessed more than one instance of poor maternal care by professionals who were overextended or who were ill suited to the caregiving role. I often heard mothers speak of feeling they had been unheard in some major or minor way during labor and delivery.

The sum of those experiences led me to develop a generally negative view on hospital birth. With that as the backdrop for my own pregnancy, I planned a home birth with a midwife whom I believed would listen and attend to my concerns. I chose this route also because I wanted to avoid routine hospital obstetric procedures that I considered unnecessarily risky. I realize that choosing that route depended on my relative advantages in terms of overall good health, supportive family members, reasonable health insurance, and access to good midwives with hospital connections. I am fully aware that many women, my own relatives and friends included, would not find such an approach acceptable for themselves, even if it were available. My own choice, however, does not correspond to wholesale opposition to hospital birth or obstetric intervention: I believe women and newborns benefit from having more rather than fewer options, and I would like to see a greater effort among obstetric professionals to fully inform mothers of their available options, including those that might be outside their scope of practice.

Study Method

Because contemporary childbirth take place in a complex context but is at the same time highly personal and individual, a case study approach (Yin, 2008) was deemed best to address questions on the match between maternal expectations and later childbirth experiences. This allowed for identifying and tracking the unique trajectories that participants' maternal expectations took from the time at which they first made them known to me in advanced pregnancy to the time of a postpartum follow-up interview.

I recruited women previously unknown to me to interview in late pregnancy and again approximately two months postpartum. Because case study research involves exploring participant views and experiences in depth, sample sizes are necessarily smaller than in traditional quantitative work (Holloway, 2008; Sandelowski, 1995). With my study focused not only on the maternal experience itself but also on the context within which it occurred, I intentionally sought women from diverse (as opposed to similar) demographic and geographic backgrounds, reflecting a criterion sampling strategy (Glaser, 1978). Balancing the interest in obtaining participant diversity with an equal interest in adequate in-depth analysis, I aimed for a sample of 75. The study received institutional ethics board approval.

From 2007 to 2009, I interviewed 82 pregnant women (expecting some attrition) in or near the third trimester of pregnancy recruited from electronic bulletin boards, regional medical clinics, and parent support organizations. Of the original 82 in the study, 75 (91.5%) completed the second interview. Mothers came from three locations: Most came from a midsize Pacific Northwestern metropolitan area and neighboring rural communities, and 20% came from either a large southern metropolitan area or a rural area in the Northeast of the United States. I interviewed about 30% of the mothers in person and the rest over the phone. Pregnancy interviews lasted 45–130 minutes, and the postpartum interviews lasted 20–90 minutes. I gave mothers a $15 retail gift card after each interview. The prenatal and postpartum interviews appear in the appendix.

My sample was not a statistical cross section of U.S. mothers, but it was diverse. Maternal education ranged from 8th grade to postgraduate, and annual family incomes ranged from no reliable income source to well above $75,000. About 30% were giving birth for the first time. Sixteen (21%) mothers were nonwhite, identifying themselves as Asian-American, African-American, Latina, or mixed race. Most mothers were married or had stable partners. Additional maternal demographic details appear in each of the individual birth-approach chapters (3–8).

I constructed a two-part, semistructured interview to elicit maternal accounts of childbirth expectations and subsequent experiences. Mothers completed the first interview during the last trimester of pregnancy and the second about two months postpartum, when childbirth-related emotions should technically have stabilized (O'Hara, 1987; Soliday, McCluskey-Fawcett, & O'Brien, 1999). Although I used the same basic set of questions with each participant, I often went "off script" to elicit more detail.

After transcribing audiotaped interviews verbatim, I applied well-established strategies for identifying themes, reducing and combining data, and validating thematic categories (Moustakas, 1994; Strauss & Corbin, 1990) in mothers' original expectations that could be compared to their subsequent experiences. Then, to provide complete images of how well maternal expectations matched their individual childbirth experiences, I reviewed each case and identified instances in which themes were confirmed or violated. Each chapter contains a general accounting of expectancy confirmation and violation, followed by representative case descriptions.

The most salient thematic categories distinguishing subgroups of mothers were their expectations of discrete birth approaches, or pathways, and I describe the discrete pathways along with information relevant to expectations in chapter 2. I cover each pathway in an individual chapter that opens with research relevant to understanding that pathway's contemporary context followed by individual cases. Chapters are roughly organized according to the percentage of mothers expecting the particular pathway, with more frequently endorsed pathways appearing first, including vaginal birth in hospital with no anticipated intervention (chapter 3), anticipated spinal (epidural) labor analgesia (chapter 4), or a "wait and see" approach to epidural analgesia (chapter 5). Less commonly pursued were planned cesarean delivery (chapter 6), vaginal birth after cesarean (VBAC; chapter 7) and out-of-hospital birth (chapter 8). Chapter 9 reviews cross-cutting themes and their implications. Within the context of my familiarity with scientific evidence on childbirth, my personal views, and my own positive personal birth experience, I found myself at times uplifted and at others saddened by what my interviewees said about their experiences—on which I focus for the remainder of the book.

ENDNOTES

1. This finding holds only when mothers are not allowed access to oral fluids, a common but outdated hospital policy; allowing mothers access to adequate fluid intake negates IV fluid effects on shortening labor duration. See Coco et al. (2010).
2. Lang and King (2008) and Hoyert (2007) have suggested that maternal mortality could be considerably higher than national statistics indicate due to limitations in current recording strategies. Also frequently overlooked in maternal mortality statistics are wide disparities in maternal death along lines of race and income.

Chapter 2

Expected Childbirth Pathways

About a century ago, when my great-grandmother was a young woman pregnant with her first child, she expected her journey from conception to delivery to involve waiting for labor to begin and enduring the experience (probably at home) for as long it took to reach its conclusion—optimally, vaginal delivery of a live newborn. Mothers of her time expected childbirth to proceed along this one and invariant conception-to-delivery pathway because none other existed, at least for the vast majority of mothers (R. W. Wertz & D. C. Wertz, 1989). In this context of limited options, mothers were the primary decision makers and agents in the birth process; nature was the primary agent in childbirth outcomes.

It is safe to say that 21st-century U.S. mothers would quickly trade childbirth of a century past for that of today, believing that contemporary birthing women and their offspring enjoy greater safety and a range of desirable options in childbirth. Greater safety is indisputable: Since 1900, infant mortality has decreased 90%, and maternal mortality has decreased 99% (United States Center for Disease Control and Prevention, 1999a). In real numbers, 6–9 women died per 1,000 live births in 1900, and by 1999, the figure had dropped to less than 0.1 per 1,000 (CDC, 1999b). In 2007, that rate translated into fewer than 1,000 U.S. maternal deaths among the more than four million live births (Xu, Kochanek, Murphy, & Tejada-Vera, 2010).

Impressive maternal mortality reductions have come almost wholly from infection control practices within institutions and by obstetric caregivers and from treatments for excessive maternal bleeding (Campbell & Graham, 2006; Loudon, 1992). In infant mortality, the role of medical advances per se remains less certain, for infant mortality corresponds closely to broad-based social indicators such as adequate nutrition, clean water, sanitation, and national income (World Bank, 1993). Regardless, most contemporary U.S. women expect to survive childbirth, and reflecting the low probability of maternal death in the 21st-century United States, only one of my interviewees directly stated mortality-related concern when revealing her expectations, saying, "It doesn't happen much anymore, but mothers die during birth sometimes, so I'd not like for that to happen!" None of my interviewees was aware of any serious risks faced by her fetus, and not a single mother mentioned concerns about newborn survival. Apparently fully expecting themselves and their offspring to survive childbirth, mothers instead framed their childbirth expectations in relationship to 21st-century childbirth pathways and obstetric options, certain components of which they anticipated would enhance childbirth safety and others they expected would enhance the quality of their experiences.

EXPECTED CHILDBIRTH PATHWAY

Social change, advanced knowledge of female anatomy and the childbirth process, and medical procedures designed to alter labor and delivery in a presumably beneficial way have resulted in multiple pathways from conception to childbirth—as opposed to the single one available to most women a century ago. Figure 1 represents anticipated childbirth pathways drawn from maternal responses to questions on their health before and during pregnancy, what they expected to happen in labor and delivery, who they anticipated would attend their birth, and whether they anticipated specific birth options from a recommended standard birth plan (Kaufman, 2007).

FIGURE 1. Expected Birth Pathways.

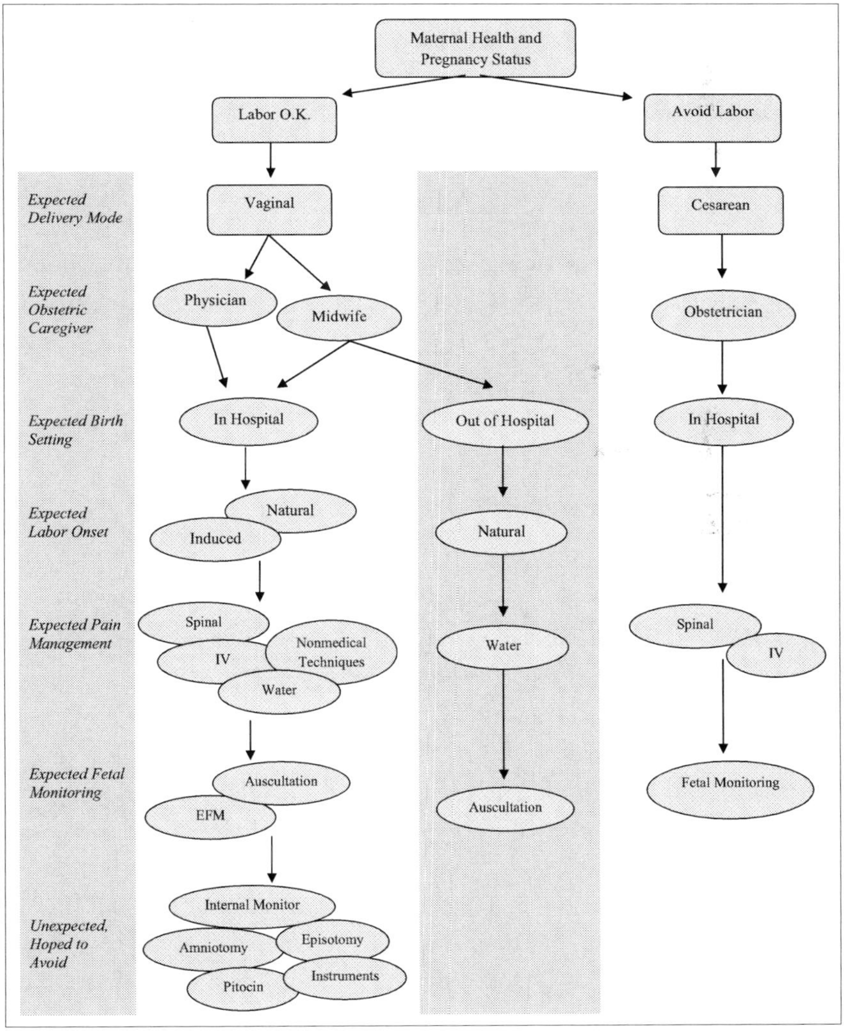

Before I proceed to the details of each step on the pathway, a few general comments are in order. First, figure 1 by no means represents exhaustive coverage of available birth options. Instead, the figure reflects those features of and options along the childbirth pathway emerging as most salient in the reported childbirth expectations of my interviewees, who were all on the verge of living out the options they envisioned. Second, this model's relatively linear structure is my own design; mothers spoke of their expectations in less circumscribed ways, and the figure represents those points they repeated or emphasized most strongly. Third, the figure's linear organization lends the impression that one expectation flowed from the one preceding it, in stepwise fashion. Although steps along the childbirth pathway should theoretically be discrete—for example, the choice of in- versus out-of-hospital birth should be independent from the choice of an obstetric caregiver—maternal accounts revealed that in reality, choices and related expectations between and among certain steps are interdependent. As a general rule, however, maternal health and pregnancy status stood as the critical point from which other expectations flowed.

Maternal and Pregnancy Status Guide Other Expectations

Setting the stage for all further expectations along the childbirth pathway was mothers' health in pregnancy and related status, a situation over which women have some, albeit limited, control. Fortunately, however, according to the World Health Organization (1996), 90–95% of pregnancies are "normal," meaning that they are free of identifiable factors known to produce adverse birth experiences or outcomes. Consistent with that figure, in initial interviews, 68 (91%) mothers described themselves as healthy or as having only minor health problems that they did not expect to complicate the labor process, defining those mothers as low risk and perhaps driving their assumptions of surviving childbirth. In theory, low-risk mothers should be able to expect to follow any one of several childbirth pathways because low-risk birth can by definition be successfully carried out in various ways.

In contrast to the theoretically open pathways in low-risk childbirth, higher risk can constrain childbirth pathways in different ways depending on individual circumstances (I use the term *higher risk* to reflect the limited predictive value of many risk factors). Seven mothers (9%) described known risk factors in their pregnancies. One mother with a history of serious kidney problems saw her choice of caregivers and subsequent steps on the pathway restricted by a referral to her community's single perinatologist; the same constraint applied to two other mothers, one with severely low amniotic fluid, the other with cervical problems. One mother had preexisting type II diabetes, and her obstetrician had forewarned her of a possible change from an anticipated spontaneous vaginal delivery pathway to induced labor or to planned cesarean. Of the 16 (21%) mothers whose status was considered too risky for labor (see the following section on delivery mode), three had an identified risk factor: Two were pregnant with twins, and one had a surgical scar that precluded safe natural labor. Thirteen mothers were restricting their delivery modes because of previous cesarean delivery in the absence of other risk factors (see chapters 6 and 7).

Expected Delivery Mode

Maternal status determined which of the two available contemporary delivery modes, vaginal or cesarean delivery, mothers might expect. Cesarean delivery can be either labored, occurring after a mother anticipating vaginal birth has labored for a time, or planned in advance of labor to avoid labor's physical stress and risks. Mothers planning cesarean anticipate surgery well ahead of time and therefore do not expect any labor experience. Standard birth-certificate reporting procedures render the breakdown between labored and planned cesarean difficult to ascertain (MacDorman, Menacker, & Declercq, 2008); however, an estimated half of the total 32% of U.S. mothers delivering by cesarean were planned because of a previous cesarean (Sakala & Corry, 2008), and "repeat cesareans" constitute by far the largest percentage of planned cesarean cases (see chapter 6). Higher risk is not necessarily cause for planned cesarean. For example, of this study's 16 (21%) mothers planning cesarean delivery, only three reported clearly identified risk factors, and the remaining mothers planning cesarean had undergone previous cesareans without other identified risk factors (see chapter 6).

Again speaking strictly theoretically, low-risk mothers anticipating vaginal birth have more flexibility in childbirth pathways than mothers expecting (planning) cesarean. For example, a low-risk mother anticipating vaginal birth can plan to give birth in or outside a hospital, whereas a mother planning cesarean delivery is constrained to, and therefore expects, hospital birth. Mothers planning VBAC are the exception for reasons discussed in chapter 7 and usually have their anticipated pathway restricted to hospital birth. Of my 75 interviewees, 59 (79%) anticipated vaginal birth; I placed them into subcategories based on their reported expectations of

- hospital birth without obstetric intervention (15, or 25%)
- hospital birth with spinal (epidural) labor analgesia (24, or 39%)
- hospital birth and "wait and see" on epidural analgesia (10, or 17%)
- hospital vaginal birth after cesarean (VBAC) without obstetric intervention (5, or 7%)
- planned out-of-hospital births with no obstetric intervention (5, or 7%).

Among the 59 mothers planning vaginal birth were three (5%) who reported identified concerns that placed them at higher risk (one planning an epidural, one "wait and see," one VBAC); the remaining 56 were low-risk mothers. Despite the various and vague terms they used to refer to the expectation of vaginal delivery—for example, *natural childbirth* to describe vaginal birth with or without expected obstetric intervention—one feature unified all study mothers anticipating vaginal delivery: With only one exception, they held an across-the-board and strongly stated desire to avoid cesarean surgery.

In contrast to vaginally birthing mothers' use of veiled language to describe their delivery mode, the 16 mothers anticipating planned cesarean delivery uniformly referred to their delivery mode as *planned cesarean* or *planned c-section*. Furthermore, their reports evidenced mixed feelings on avoiding labor and vaginal birth, with four (25%) mothers expressing some ambivalence about their anticipated childbirth pathway. Two of those four equivocated on the decision, referring, for example, to difficulty deciding between planned cesarean or VBAC, or mentioning resentment over perceived pressure from medical professionals to decide. The other two mothers planning cesarean delivery said they definitely would have preferred vaginal birth but "could not" pursue this approach because of either a convincing medical recommendation or an institutional policy. The remaining mothers in this group expressed no particular enthusiasm or excitement about the upcoming birth process, but they did comment on the advantage of knowing what to expect by virtue of either a previous cesarean birth or what they presumed would be a straightforward surgical procedure.

Expected Obstetric Caregiver in Birth

With surgical training and practice primary features distinguishing physician from nonphysician obstetric caregivers, 15 of the 16 mothers anticipating cesarean delivery expected that an obstetrician would attend their births specifically to perform the surgery; one mother unfamiliar with obstetric training and practice was unsure whether a midwife or an obstetrician would perform surgery. Similarly, in the wake of professional recommendations for planned VBAC care (ACOG, 2010), all mothers planning VBAC expected to have an obstetrician attend their births.

Because mothers anticipating vaginal delivery are not planning surgery, nonphysician obstetric caregivers (certified midwives or nurse-midwives, in the present case) may theoretically attend non-VBAC vaginal births in or outside hospitals. Of the 59 mothers planning vaginal birth (including VBAC), 32 anticipated a physician-attended birth (30 obstetricians, 2 family practice physicians), and 22 anticipated either an available midwife or physician obstetric caregiver. All five mothers anticipating midwife-attended births were in the out-of-hospital subgroup.

Although many associate midwives with no- or low-intervention birth, only about half the mothers who saw midwives for their prenatal care anticipated intervention-free natural childbirth and, correspondingly, anticipated having the birth possibly attended by a midwife (the alternative being an obstetrician). In contrast, some mothers who anticipated technological birth intervention received only midwife care during pregnancy with the expectation of having an obstetrician-attended birth. For example, Iris expected an obstetrician-attended birth with an epidural but had met only with nurse-midwives in prenatal appointments. Sharon, planning cesarean delivery, said, "I've been seeing a nurse-midwife ... However, because we do know I have to have a c-section ... my care will be handled by an OB/GYN who is able to actually do the cesarean section when that time comes."

Consistent with national statistics showing that physicians attend about 93% of hospital births (Martin et al., 2010), only one among the dozen hospital-birthing mothers who had purposely sought midwife care in pregnancy anticipated with certainty a midwife-attended hospital birth. Moreover, only 10 (13%) of this study's 75 mothers anticipated that a prenatal care provider known to them would attend their births: One mother had sought the only physician in her area who would agree to attend VBAC, one "wait and see" mother scheduled labor induction, and another switched from planned VBAC to planned cesarean to meet preferred physician availability; the two mothers of twins also planned cesarean delivery around their preferred physicians' input and availability. The remaining five mothers anticipating the same caregiver across pregnancy and delivery were planning midwife-attended home birth; four of those stated that continuous caregiving had partly motivated their out-of-hospital birth decisions, as in Carla's statement, "I wanted ... more personal one-on-one care with someone I knew throughout the entire pregnancy."

To give mothers at least an opportunity to meet those who might attend their birth, clinics may intentionally rotate prenatal-care patients among clinic staff, and about half this study's mothers referred to having experienced such practices. For example, Ana, planning cesarean delivery, said, "I'm in a clinic with other doctors and nurse-midwives … I meet each one of them … depending on the scheduling … I don't decide, they decide for me." Echoing a similar lack of control over clinic practices designed to improve continuity of care, Heidi, planning natural birth in a hospital, said, "They work as a team, [and] I had a different one [provider] every month … a team wasn't my choice; that's how they do it."

In contrast to the small percentage of mothers who could actually count on a specific obstetric caregiver, over 90% of the total sample said they felt it was at least somewhat important for them to know their obstetric caregiver in advance, echoing what Tasha (planning cesarean birth) said: "She [the obstetrician] knows me, rather than having a stranger do it." Despite this preference for a continuous caregiver from pregnancy to delivery, most mothers expected and had accepted that they had little choice in the matter—in one first-time mother's words, "It may not be her [midwife] when I have the baby, I understand," or, stated more firmly by this second-time mother, "I think it's important, but I know it's not going to happen." There were, however, exceptions: Iris (planning an epidural) declared, "I don't care. As long as they know what they're doing, I'm fine"; similarly, in-hospital natural-birthing mother Elise said, "I'd rather have a healthy baby."

Expected Birth Setting

A mother's choice of birth setting, broadly distinguished as in-hospital versus out-of-hospital birth, depends first on pregnancy status, with out-of-hospital birth generally restricted to lower risk mothers (e.g., ACOG, 2011b; Wax, Pinette, & Cartin, 2010). In addition, maternal decisions on and related expectations for obstetric caregivers and birth settings are interdependent because most caregivers limit their practices to one setting or the other. For example, birth-setting options for my interviewee Aisha, who felt close to her obstetrician, were constrained because that obstetrician practiced only in hospitals. In planned cesarean, a mother's decision and expectation for birth setting is implicit because nonemergency cesarean surgery (generally) occurs only in fully equipped, traditional hospital obstetric units; reflecting that assumption, none of this study's 16 mothers anticipating planned cesarean made explicit mention of birth setting in relationship to her expectations.

In contrast and at least technically, low-risk mothers like those 54 non-VBAC, vaginally birthing mothers in my sample, could freely choose between giving birth in a hospital or in another nonhospital setting. The choice of birth setting subsequently opens (or closes) additional options and feeds into distinct maternal expectations. With nearly 99% of contemporary mothers birthing in hospitals (Martin et al., 2010), expecting hospital birth seems almost automatic. With the prevailing cultural view of hospital birth as the normative and safest place for childbirth, a mother who decides to "opt out" risks hearing from others that she is jeopardizing her own or her offspring's well-being (Lothian, 2001). Of my interviewees, 70 (93%) expected hospital birth—by far the majority of my sample but lower than the national rate.

Among those low-risk mothers anticipating hospital birth, nearly all began describing their childbirth expectations without explicitly stating that they had chosen this birth setting, in line with the cultural expectation of hospital birth. Two first-time mothers directly echoed the prevailing cultural belief that hospital birth offers safety and comfort in stating why they *had* chosen hospital birth. Rebecca said, "I just feel like it's smarter for me to work in a more medical setting, and I feel more at peace about that so it keeps me a little more calm." And this was echoed by Bella:

> For this being my first child, there is something really comforting about being in a hospital and knowing that I'll have nurses there to like help me figure out what to do with the baby 'cause I really don't know what I'm doing.

Only one mother planning hospital birth explicitly stated a negative view of the hospital setting, saying, "It seems that every time I go, someone I know is dying."

The few hospital-birthing mothers who, unprompted, mentioned anything about expecting to give birth in hospitals referred to why they *had not* chosen out-of-hospital birth, and external influences—rather than personal preferences—were the deciding factor. For example, Gillian said her first hospital birth had gone so easily that she would "rather give birth at home," but her husband "couldn't live with it, if something happened." Aisha also would have preferred to "set it up at home" because she had multiple pets that needed "kept an eye on." Lydia cited financial restrictions, saying, "I might have been more open to doing a home birth, but home births are more expensive and they're not covered by insurance." Lydia's statements on the higher costs of home birth reflect wider cultural misinformation on obstetric care expenditures: Reliable estimates place the average home-birth cost at 68% less than uncomplicated vaginal delivery in a hospital (R. E. Anderson & D. A. Anderson, 1999), though costs may vary as a function of the home-birth attendant's credentials and hospital procedures used (Henderson & Petrou, 2008). However, underscoring the lack of cultural acceptance of home birth as generally safe, many insurers do not cover home-birth costs.

The five mothers anticipating out-of-hospital birth explicitly mentioned birth setting in describing their expectations. Like the decisions of mothers planning cesarean delivery, mothers' decisions to deliver at home were inseparable from the desire for a particular obstetric caregiver who they believed would support natural birth and whom they had observed attending a birth or in whose abilities they had full confidence. For example, Melinda said of her midwife, "My sister has used her for all her births. I knew her personally before. I grew up with her daughters … [The midwives are] very calm, very trustworthy, very experienced." Along similar lines, Ginger said, "My sister actually used her [the midwife]. And I was present at my sister's birth and I just really liked her, so we went with her."

Expected Labor and Delivery Companions

Every mother in my study expected someone close to her to provide support, company, or advocacy during childbirth. All mothers with a committed partner or spouse expected the partners to accompany them throughout labor and delivery, except one mother whose spouse was overseas. That mother and the small number of mothers without committed partners or spouses expected a sibling, a close friend, or other family member to accompany them. Fifteen mothers expected additional company in birth from their own mothers, mothers-in-law, siblings, or a friend who happened to be a trained doula (birth support person). Four mothers anticipated having to turn family members away from accompanying them in hospital birth. The specific support functions mothers expected of their labor and delivery companions varied from acting as a supportive presence to outright advocacy—for instance, "My husband is totally on board with my wishes, and in case I can't make them known and if there's too many people around or they're trying to interfere ... he will stand up."

EXPECTED LABOR ONSET

Because planned cesarean birth is designed to circumvent the labor process, 15 of the16 mothers planning this childbirth pathway shared an expectation of no labor onset, but one mother expecting twins suspected that she might go into labor prematurely. Most (57) of the 59 mothers anticipating vaginal birth expected spontaneous labor onset. Of those 57, two said they suspected their labor would ultimately be induced because they had had labor induced in a previous birth. Two other mothers had scheduled labor induction for a day on or near their due dates; one mother stated that the reason for this decision was that her labor had been induced previously and her physician did not want her to go "too late," and the other said that her midwife had agreed to schedule induction to avoid the fetus's growing overly large. Although few mothers expected labor induction, the overall sentiment towards labor induction was decidedly mixed among the remaining mothers anticipating vaginal delivery: Naturally birthing and VBAC mothers generally expressed the view that induction was unnecessary if not harmful; some but not all mothers in the two epidural groups expressed readier acceptance of labor induction primarily out of concerns about large fetal size.

Labor induction may involve oral medications, vaginal inserts, and perhaps most familiar to mothers, IV administration of hormones. The 21st century's 41% labor induction rate (up from 1.1% in 1980; Declercq et al., 2006; DeFrances et al., 2007) is considerably higher than the World Health Organization and Pan American Health Organization's (1985) recommended optimal rate of 10%. Recent ACOG practice guidelines state that "indications for labor induction are not absolute" (2009, p. 389), leaving the door open to more inductions. An estimated one third of today's inductions are performed for one of several proposed medical reasons, and the other two thirds are performed without identified medical cause, or as "elective" inductions (Caughey et al., 2009). Controversy surrounds labor induction's effects on the birth process, which include associated higher rates of additional obstetric intervention and cesarean birth (Moleti, 2009; Ramsey, Ramin, & Ramin, 2000), as well as the effects of artificially shortening human gestational age (Sakala, 2006).

Expected Childbirth Pain Relief

Fifteen of the 16 mothers planning cesarean birth confirmed the expectation of pain relief as a component in their expected childbirth pathways only when prompted. Reflecting the general faith mothers put in cesarean delivery's anesthetic procedures, one mother said, "I just have to watch an orderly administer it ... I don't have to go through any of that type of pain or pushing." Only one planned cesarean mother raised an unprompted concern over childbirth pain while revealing her childbirth expectations, saying she anticipated pain despite her obstetrician's reassurance that she would receive effective medical pain relief. Nearly all mothers in this group expected postpartum pain but also that pain medication would effectively reduce it.

Because they are not anticipating major surgery, vaginally birthing mothers theoretically have full flexibility to choose which, if any, medical or nonmedical pain-relief strategies they might desire and whether and when to formalize their wishes. Specific childbirth pain-relief strategies were a primary defining feature of three (four, including out-of-hospital births) vaginally birthing subgroups: 100% of hospital natural and out-of-hospital birthing mothers expressed no expectation of, no desire for, and opposition to pain medication (their reasons varied; see chapters 3 and 8); 100% of mothers anticipating pain medication made their wishes known to obstetric caregivers in advance; 100% of mothers in the "wait and see" group said they accepted epidural administration as a viable option but preferred to decide on it only after having labored for a time.

Mothers in the out-of-hospital and hospital-natural-birth subgroups further distinguished themselves by expecting to use (or not to use) nonmedical pain-relief techniques. Three hospital-natural-birth mothers reported having practiced established pain relief techniques that they expected would help them cope with the intense pain they anticipated. For example, Simone said she practiced deep breathing techniques she learned about from media and professionals, and after reading about birth hypnosis, Bella purchased home-study materials and practiced the techniques. One out-of-hospital and five hospital-natural-birth mothers said they had not practiced specific pain-relief strategies but that they did anticipate having birth tubs available for nonmedical pain relief. All this group's mothers expected that the water would help them effectively manage pain, expressing the general belief that water would help them avoid an unwanted epidural.

I should point out that *epidural* is an umbrella term used in reference to several anesthetic procedures used to deliver pain medication directly into the spinal column (see chapter 4), and that epidurals may be used for a variety of medical indications beyond obstetrics, such as chronic back pain and orthopedic surgery. For the sake of readability, I use the term *epidural* along with appropriate descriptors as the material warrants. Constituting the majority of vaginally birthing mothers, 34 (56%) of my interviewees either anticipated having an epidural or were open to one if labor warranted it. Though figures on how many mothers plan for an epidural (as opposed to receiving it during the course of labor) are not readily available, one study on expectant mothers with birth plans—a select group—indicated that approximately 62% expressly opposed epidural in advance of labor, and the remaining 38% were either open to epidural or had planned on having it (Deering, Zaret, McGaha & Satin, 2007). Across the nation, reported obstetric epidural administration rates range from 49% for Hispanic mothers to 69% for non-Hispanic white mothers (Osterman, 2009), with wide variability depending on maternal age, race, and U.S. region.

From a psychological perspective, planning epidural administration allows mothers to expect help with labor pain shortly upon hospital arrival because the planning would allow them to look forward to what they believed would be effective pain relief and to obtaining it in a timely fashion. Speaking both to the benefits she anticipated from advance planning of an epidural and to her expectations of its effectiveness, first-time mother Iris said, "I'm probably wrong; in my mind, I'm not worried about it [childbirth]. Epidural, and I'm fine." Another first-time mother expected only limited pain, saying she believed that after having her epidural administered, labor would consist primarily of "a lot of waiting." As further evidence of the trust advance-planning mothers placed in epidural pain relief, four stated no interest in learning about nonmedical pain relief strategies; one 25-year-old mother stated that she "didn't pay attention to" talk of nonmedical strategies in her childbirth classes because she planned to "just get the epidural."

Mothers in the "wait and see" group were similarly convinced of epidural analgesia's pain-reducing potential but, wanting some sense of whether they would perceive the need for a procedure before formalizing any commitment to it, expected to labor for a time without it. One first-time mother said, "I'm keeping it as an option because I've never done this before, and I don't know what it will be like." After having an epidural that she had planned with her first birth, one mother recalled that the procedure slowed her labor and made it "hard to know when to push," so she preferred to attempt her second labor medication-free before committing to the procedure. Another mother said along similar lines, "I don't know what I'm going to do … [I'm] trying not to set too many standards." In expecting to "wait and see," maternal control over if and when to request the procedure is, theoretically, tempered by less control over the availability of an anesthesiology professional to perform it on request.

Maternal expectations varied across groups about receiving another widely used pain relief option, systemic analgesia—usually opiate medications administered orally, by an injection, or by IV to produce a "total body" effect (Hinova & Fernando, 2009). Mothers in the naturally birthing groups said they neither expected systemic opiates nor found them acceptable; none of the mothers in either epidural group said they expected systemic opiates but would find them acceptable if circumstances warranted it. Mothers in the planned cesarean group expected some sort of systemic pain relief but were unsure whether that would occur during or after the surgery.

In theory, systemic opiates are administered in low enough doses to dampen overall pain sensation but leave a mother sufficiently alert to participate in the birth process; effects vary widely (Hinova & Fernando, 2009). With an understanding of how opiates work and the ability to control dosage and administration, professionals consider systemic analgesia in childbirth generally safe. However, concerns have been raised over systemic opiates' variable effectiveness and their effects on the fetus: Opiate drugs cross the placenta and enter the fetus's system, and some studies have indicated slowed fetal heart rate in labor, reduced neonatal responsiveness, and early breastfeeding problems as possible consequences (Reynolds, 2010).

Expected Maternal and Fetal Monitoring

Contemporary childbirth almost always involves use of basic or highly advanced techniques to assess the status of two patients, the mother and fetus, for whom mothers and their obstetric caregivers must ultimately make decisions. Across subgroups, no mother mentioned any expectation of routine monitoring of *maternal* status, such as blood loss or vital signs (including blood pressure, heart rate, and body temperature). Mothers did, however, report expecting some form of fetal monitoring, with experienced mothers uniformly expecting it and about half of first-time mothers mentioning any such expectation without prompting.

In contemporary practice, over 85% of 21st-century hospital births involve electronic fetal monitoring (EFM), most commonly continuous fetal cardiotocography (CTG), a noninvasive procedure requiring that the mother lie still on her back with a flexible belt strapped to her abdomen; the belt transmits maternal and fetal data to a printer. Introduced in the 1960s, CTG was expected to reduce birth-related brain damage and quickly began replacing auscultation (listening to fetal heart beat with a stethoscope). Over the years, CTG has aroused controversy in part because anticipated drops in neonatal brain damage or fetal deaths have not corresponded to its use (Alfirevic, Devane, & Gyte, 2006), likely because the sometimes ambiguous data it yields defy straightforward interpretation (U.S. National Institute of Child Health and Human Development Research Planning Workshop, 1997). With ambiguous results in hand, physicians may be more likely to recommend intervention as a safeguard; this may perhaps explain why operative vaginal (with forceps or vacuum) and cesarean delivery occur up to twice as often in CTG compared to auscultation groups (Grivell, Alfirevic, Gyte, & Devane, 2010; Steer, 2008). Invasive internal fetal monitoring procedures requiring intravaginal insertion of medical devices yield more accurate results and are associated with fewer subsequent interventions, but those involving incisions in the fetal scalp significantly raise infection risk (Chourasia & Tiwani, 2008; Mozurkewich & Wolf, 2000). Mothers generally find internal fetal monitoring procedures aversive because they always involve extra vaginal exams and manipulation for placement of monitoring devices and often require an incision in the fetus's scalp to place an electrode in the "pocket" created by the incision.

Of the two mothers who, without prompting, expressed an expectation of fetal monitoring during labor, both were naturally birthing, one in and the other outside the hospital, and both described fetal monitoring (electronic and manual, respectively) as something they looked forward to and appreciated. Once prompted, however, all the experienced and about half the first-time vaginally birthing mothers said they anticipated some form of fetal monitoring. All out-of-hospital birthing mothers expected auscultation, whereas only two planning vaginal birth in the hospital expected it. The remaining hospital mothers anticipating vaginal birth alluded directly or indirectly to EFM (e.g., "the belt thingy"). These same mothers seemed to accept EFM as routine and as beneficial in its potential to reassure—for example, "It's cool … a great way to know how your baby's doing." Third-time mother Amanda said, "It's nice to know that the baby is OK … it's nice for reassuring … to know that things are going well from the baby's point of view." One first-time mother said she assumed EFM had some benefit but that she did not "really understand why they do it." Other mothers resented EFM's imposed limitations on their movement; one said that she did not like to be "hooked up to all kinds of machines."

When asked specifically about internal monitoring, most vaginally birthing mothers said they "didn't know" whether to expect it and had no further opinion on the matter. Only two mothers, both experienced, said that they "didn't care" whether it was used or that they would readily accept it "if necessary." Three others expressed varying degrees of opposition: Second-time mother Amy said, "I'm not sure how well that actually works," and two mothers took a firm stand against internal (but not external) monitoring, both having had previous negative experiences. Kate said she had written her opposition to internal monitoring into her birth plan because "they did that with my son, and I didn't want it again." Similarly, another experienced mother said, "We would not allow that." All mothers planning cesarean delivery assumed that some form of fetal monitoring would be used during surgery but none named a specific procedure.

WHAT MOTHERS EXPECTED TO AVOID UNLESS "MEDICALLY NECESSARY"

According to national statistics on hospital obstetric-procedure practice rates, mothers can reasonably expect procedures well beyond those discussed thus far. With that prior knowledge, I anticipated that the following procedures would become part of some of my interviewees' experiences, but with my emphasis on *their* expectations, I prompted mothers by asking whether they anticipated having any of the following interventions. With a few exceptions noted throughout, primiparous and multiparous mothers generally could not say whether they anticipated specific birth procedures apart from epidural administration. However, most mothers added that they preferred not to have such procedures but would undergo them "if medically necessary" or if fetal well-being somehow depended on it.

Labor Acceleration

In the present-day United States, a pervasive and chronic sense of time pressure and time shortage characterizes the culture at large (Robinson & Godbey, 2005); thus, it should come as little surprise that the obstetric profession operates in parallel, placing intense focus on the timing and duration of specific events on the path from labor onset to delivery. Medical techniques designed to keep mothers on a predetermined labor-to-delivery time course are collectively referred to as "labor acceleration procedures." Most of these practices come from Irish obstetrician Dr. Kieran O'Driscoll's 1968 "active labor management" treatment protocol (program) designed to reduce the emotional and physical stress he had observed in the handful of first-time mothers who experienced prolonged first-stage labors, up to 36 hours in some cases (Boylan, 1989). Called *active labor management* for medical staff's active role in continuously supporting laboring women, the original program involved (1) educating mothers on hospital care, (2) admitting them to the hospital only after labor had technically begun, (3) amniotomy (breaking of the membranes) to test for the safety of administering oxytocin (a hormone to speed labor up), (4) administering oxytocin only when labor has slowed, and (5) ensuring continuous presence of a nurse or midwife to record maternal emotional and physical state. When practiced in this form, active labor management has been shown to shorten first-stage labor duration by 2–5 hours (Brown, Paranjothy, Dowswell, &

Thomas, 2008; Frigoletto et al., 1995) and to reduce childbirth fever (Frigoletto et al., 1995).

According to Boylan (1989), active labor management has become confused with aggressive obstetric intervention, whereas the original O'Driscoll program was designed and shown to reduce obstetric intervention through the active *supervision* of labor by physicians and through the reassurance provided by nurses continuously present with mothers throughout labor. Unfortunately, it is difficult to track how many U.S. institutions routinely practice the all-important continuous nurse presence component of active labor management because standard national data reporting protocols do not contain this variable. Based on available data, however, the term *active* in the U.S. hospital context appears to have become synonymous with aggressive labor acceleration and aggressive medical intervention (Pates & Satin, 2005). For example, amniotomy was rarely performed in 1980 (in only about 3.2% of cases; DeFrances et al., 2007), whereas 59% of mothers giving birth in 2006 had amniotomy (Declercq et al., 2006). Alongside widespread practice of amniotomy has emerged a good deal of controversy over its risks, including its potential to stall labor progress, to intensify pain, and to increase infection risk. Its benefits in helping labor progress more quickly have been difficult to establish because no firm standards on appropriate timing of the procedure have been developed (Smyth, Alldred, & Markham, 2007; Stewart, Kennedy & Calder, 1982; Vincent, 2005; Wei et al., 2009).

Oxytocin administration has steadily increased in recent years, with a threefold jump from 17.4% of mothers in 1997 to 55% in 2006 (Declercq et al., 2006; Wei, Luo, Xu, & Fraser, 2009). Oxytocin works gradually, and its effects vary markedly between individuals; improper dosing can produce dangerous consequences (Alfirevic, Kelly, & Dowswell, 2009). For these reasons, the Institute for Safe Medication Practices put synthetic oxytocin on its "high alert" list, which currently contains 11 other drugs with similarly dangerous potential (Clark, Simpson, Knox, & Garite, 2009). In the words of one team of obstetricians, "We know of no other area in medicine in which a potentially dangerous drug is administered to hasten completion of a physiologic process that would, if left to its own devices, usually complete itself without incurring the risk of drug administration" (Clark et al., 2009, p. 35e.3). Reflecting my interviewees' across-the-board preference to avoid oxytocin, one second-time mother said, "I hate it; that's nasty stuff."

Episiotomy

Any discussion of mothers' expectations about vaginal birth and their resultant experiences would be incomplete without mention of episiotomy, a surgical cut (usually) from the posterior end of the vaginal opening toward the anus, pioneered centuries ago to prevent tears surrounding the vaginal opening. The widened opening allows the obstetric caregiver to manipulate fetal shoulders that may be wedged into the birth canal (shoulder dystocia), to ease a large baby through the vaginal opening, or to more safely use forceps or vacuum extraction (Carroli & Mignini, 2009). As with many procedures introduced into early 20th-century U.S. obstetrics, episiotomy was routinely practiced well before research had been conducted on its long-term effects. By the 1960s, nearly 100% of birthing mothers had episiotomies. As studies emerged showing that episiotomy's negative effects, such as anal sphincter injury, outweighed benefits of performing the procedure without a specific medical reason, rates declined to about 30–40% of all U.S. births (with some offset owing to increased cesarean delivery), a figure many believe is still unnecessarily high.

On the lack of scientifically demonstrated benefits of episiotomy and its association with long-term problems, such as fecal and urinary incontinence, genital pain, and pain during intercourse, a past president of the American Gynecological and Obstetrical Society stated, "Rarely has a surgical procedure been performed by so many so often with so little evidence to support its widespread use" (Mueller-Heubach, 2007, p. 368). Though I cannot be certain whether my interviewees were aware of this professional obstetric perspective, I can say that of the vaginally birthing mothers in my study, none reported during pregnancy any expectation of episiotomy, though about one quarter, some of those first-time mothers, anticipated minor natural tears with vaginal delivery. Most mothers strongly opposed episiotomy. Correspondingly, two mothers, both of whom had had previous negative experiences with episiotomy, said that they had made their preferences known in advance. For example, second-time mother Georgia reported, "Last time I had an episiotomy, and they didn't really tell me they were doing it … I was concerned about it, and I did talk to my doctor about it."

Instrumental Assistance

One of vaginal birth's final steps is expulsion of the fetus through the vaginal opening, and among other things, shoulder dystocia, large fetal size, or maternal exhaustion can complicate the process. Instruments, forceps or a vacuum, may be employed but typically only as a last option. Practiced in 1–5% of all vaginal births, vacuum and forceps use has declined considerably over past decades, primarily because of physicians' lack of comfort with the technical aspects of and perceived personal liability associated with the procedures, particularly in comparison to cesarean delivery (Powell, Gilo, Foote, Gil, & Lavin, 2007). Yet when used correctly, forceps delivery carries much lower maternal mortality risk than cesarean surgery and rarely causes severe damage to mothers or fetuses (Murphy & Koh, 2007; Murphy, Liebling, Verity, Swingler, & Patel, 2001; Towner, Castro, Eby-Wilkens, & Gilbert, 1999). Vacuum assistance, involving placing a cup on the fetus's head to produce a tight vacuum seal and manually applying suction force to gently ease the fetal head out the vaginal opening (Ali & Norwitz, 2009), causes even fewer problems for mothers and is used 3–4 times more frequently than forceps (Caughey et al., 2005; Johanson et al., 1999). However, vacuum-assisted delivery can produce scalp bruising severe enough to lead to shock; over a four-year period, the U.S. Food and Drug Administration (FDA) estimated that vacuum extraction caused 12 neonatal deaths and 9 serious injuries (Bahl, Patel, Swingler, Ellis, & Murphy, 2007), leading to an FDA public health advisory on cautious use of the procedure (United States Department of Health and Human Services, FDA, 1998).

In a culture characterized by growing acceptance of cesarean delivery as a normative birth option, public health warnings against instrumental assistance in vaginal birth, and an apparent corresponding lack of widespread information on cesarean risks to mothers and newborns, I found it unsurprising that not one of my interviewees anticipating vaginal birth expected instruments to be used along the pathway to delivery. Furthermore, mothers expressed generally negative views towards instruments, not even endorsing their use "if necessary." Consistent with physicians' generally greater comfort with cesarean delivery compared to instrumental assistance, however, several mothers made known their acceptance of cesarean delivery if the situation warranted it; in Stacey's words, "I have heard about that [instrumental delivery] and I personally would not want that at all. I heard it makes the baby's head look bad. If it came to that, I would rather have c-section."

Summary and Implications

Mothers' expected birth setting, delivery mode, obstetric caregiver, labor and delivery companion(s), and pain-relief strategies (or choice to avoid them) varied, as did the relative influence on those expectations of pregnancy status, a mother's own conscious decision making, and outside factors. Theoretically, mothers with low-risk pregnancy status could construct and anticipate individual childbirth pathways from the full range of available options, whereas some mothers' statuses directed them towards a pathway with limited options—for example, planned cesarean birth. Figure 1 reflects the relative breadth of options for mothers anticipating vaginal birth in hospitals compared to women anticipating out-of-hospital birth or planned cesarean surgery. Any one study mother's expected childbirth pathway and related option set involved interdependent choices that were self-limiting, reflected in, for example, interdependence among birth setting, cultural norms, obstetric caregivers, and pain relief options.

Davis-Floyd (2001; 2004) has described three major and distinct orientations in maternal medical care. Although practice orientations vary from institution to institution and are continuously evolving, hospital birth in the United States has long been rooted in a *technocratic* medical paradigm that is slow to change and involves (among other things) practitioner-centered care and aggressive intervention to ensure desired short-term outcomes—in short, high-tech, low-touch care. The more contemporary *humanistic* model involves balanced consideration of institutional and individual needs, shared medical decision making, and compassion-driven care, or high-tech, high-touch; the *holistic* model relies on treating the whole person in a comforting context with some reliance on intuition to identify and treat problems, or low-tech, high-touch. Davis-Floyd argued that blending these approaches would result in the best maternal care possible (2001).

In describing their expectations for labor and delivery, my interviewees reflected their own blending of these care orientations. For example, across delivery modes, most mothers wanted the feeling of comfort and safety they believed a technologically advanced hospital setting offered, yet they also wanted (though did not expect) to know the person providing their birth care, a desire more aligned with a humanistic or holistic approach. Some mothers expected medical pain-relief strategies associated with a technocratic approach but reflected the shared decision-making component of humanistic maternal care in deciding whether and when to make their pain-relief desires known. The very expectation of planned out-of-hospital birth reflects a holistic orientation, although by choosing certified midwives or nurse midwives, mothers on this pathway reflected a technocratically based valuing of the benefits of a formally trained and credentialed professional obstetric caregiver.

Evidenced in rising rates of obstetric interventions with questionable benefits, particularly labor acceleration and planned cesarean delivery solely because a mother has already had one, the prevailing U.S. technocratic model of maternal care lags somewhat behind what seemed to be mothers' unique and individualized expected childbirth pathways, which involved blending distinct maternal-care orientations. The apparent mismatch between mothers' individualized views on obstetric care and contemporary technocratic, institutional maternal-care design and practices places women at high risk for having their expectations violated. Figure 1 shows that from the maternal perspective, that risk may be greatest for mothers anticipating vaginal birth in hospitals.

To clarify, taken at face value, anticipated vaginal birth involved multiple options for meeting expectations at each step of the pathway, including options for determining anticipated birth setting, obstetric caregiver in birth, and pain-relief strategies. Though for the most part mothers had developed expectations at each step—a process consistent with a humanistic orientation on patient-centered care—the dominance of the technocratic model in contemporary obstetric care could very well interfere with such expectations. In particular, a hospital-birthing mother's expectation of obtaining certain technocratic components (e.g., an epidural) but not others (e.g., what some described as unwanted, aversive internal monitoring) seems to hold particularly high risk of being violated.

In contrast, and again only on the surface, mothers operating either fully within the technocratic model, as in a planned cesarean delivery, or well outside it, as in an out-of-hospital birth, have decidedly fewer choices along the childbirth pathway and correspondingly fewer points at which their expectations may go awry. Planned cesarean delivery involves virtually no question of whether a physician will attend the birth, of whether labor induction, medical pain relief, episiotomy, or instrumental assistance will be involved, or—obviously—of whether cesarean birth will become part of the birth experience. In other words, once a mother says yes to and anticipates planned cesarean, she says yes to a total, all-inclusive technocratic care package. Along similar lines, mothers expecting out-of-hospital birth have nearly the same limited options available to mothers of a century past: They hold no expectation of induced labor, labor acceleration procedures, or electronic fetal monitoring. Of course, cesarean delivery is major surgery requiring a high level of practitioner skill and institutional support, with its own potential for unanticipated turns. Likewise, out-of-hospital birthing mothers face the prospect of unanticipated turns, though primarily in physical, rather than artificially induced, aspects of the process.

In voicing their expectations of childbirth overall, however, all mothers in this study seemed to anticipate surviving the process along with their offspring, distinguishing themselves from mothers of a century ago and allowing them to focus on the quality of the experience. How their lived experiences matched both their individual expectations and those expectations characteristic of the pathway more generally is detailed in the remaining chapters.

Chapter 3

Expectations and Experiences of Planned Hospital Natural Childbirth

The Context of Hospital Natural Childbirth

Interview question: *What does "natural childbirth" mean to you?*

Mother 1: "Vaginal birth."

Mother 2: "No c-section."

Mother 3: "I think of water birth, no epidural, no medication, just all natural."

Maternal responses to my interview question reflect how U.S. mothers today, even those seeking so-called natural childbirth, generally fail to include mention of where they anticipate giving birth. Seen in the over 99% of U.S. women in the 21st century who deliver in hospitals (Martin, Hamilton, & Sutton, 2009), hospital birth is the default, departing from the general cultural expectation of a midwife-attended home birth that prevailed among U.S. women a century ago. In the early 20th century, physicians, whose primary obstetric training consisted of the few births they had overseen, generally attended only wealthy women. In the absence of knowledge on normal birth processes, infection control, and maternal bleeding, early 20th century physicians used novel interventions that often led to disastrous results and an associated higher maternal mortality among the wealthy women they served (Loudon, 1992).

Even so, as has been true across human history, some home births presented complications beyond even the most competent midwife's ability to manage, and families began calling upon community doctors to help. For efficiency's sake, physicians gradually moved toward treating women of all social groups in hospitals, where they could systematically intervene with more patients using procedures such as twilight birth (general anesthesia to eliminate pain and erase mothers' childbirth memories, a procedure that later proved dangerous and ineffective; Arms, 1975; Epstein, 2010). With infant mortality up to 30% in some U.S. regions in the early 20th century (Lee, 2007; Lee, Paneth, Gartner, Pearlman, & Gruss, 1980), physicians were well positioned to gain community trust in professionally supervised hospital birth as superior to and safer than the home-based alternative.

Unfortunately, hospital birth could not counter the forces of intractable urban poverty, which was as much responsible for infant mortality as where or with whom women delivered their infants (Cone, 1979; Luke, Williams, Minogue, & Keith, 1993). Also unfortunately, hospital birth in the early days led to more rather than fewer maternal deaths (Loudon, 1987, 1992). Until discoveries surrounding germs as the cause of life-threatening maternal infections became accepted and translated into routine sanitary practice some time later, medical staff increased infection risk as they transmitted blood and fluids from one hospital patient to the next without stopping to attend to their own hygiene. Similar resistance to emerging knowledge on safely and effectively treating maternal hemorrhage delayed widespread uptake of simple, life-sparing practices. With livelihoods at stake, as were the desire for medical progress and the respect of a public that looked to medical professionals for solutions, the medical community kept quiet about maternal treatment and related mortality on those early obstetric wards; moreover, U.S. culture of a century ago was perhaps unready to receive revelations of suboptimal hospital obstetric care.

To say that the medical community was entirely responsible for this early and troubling phase of U.S. obstetric history would, however, be inaccurate. Operating on the early 20th-century American psyche was the powerful influence of industrialization: the medical community eagerly adopted technological and pharmacological advances as wholly beneficial, and so did the public. Specially designed obstetric facilities staffed with medical "experts" and gadgets made families think of a future made easier and brighter with science, whereas home birth seemed painfully outdated. Population dispersal offered a perfect opportunity for locating new, physician-directed maternal medical facilities.

By the middle of the 20th century, nearly half of U.S. mothers gave birth under physician supervision in hospitals (Curtin & Park, 1999; Martin et al., 2009; United States National Center for Health Statistics, 1999). I have not formally interviewed women who gave birth during that era, but reports abound of amphetamines prescribed to treat "excessive" pregnancy weight gain, mothers strapped to gurneys during their hours of labor, and general anesthesia administered without consent (Schultz, 1958). In the 1950s, too, thousands of pregnant U.S. women underwent pelvic X-ray to identify those who might need cesarean surgery. After discovering that X-ray was ineffective and suspecting that it might cause childhood leukemia (Granroth, 1979), the U.S. Food and Drug Administration (FDA) in 1981 issued a statement on limiting the procedure. In that same era, diethylstilbestrol (DES) was touted as a miracle drug to prevent miscarriages in women who had previously had several, triggering across-the-board use as a preventive measure. After learning that DES caused serious reproductive problems and cancers in users' female offspring and some risks to male offspring as well, the FDA in 1971 banned the drug (Rubin, 2007; Veurink & de Jong-van den Berg, 2005).

Reports of midcentury obstetric practices act not only as reminders of what our foremothers endured but also as indicators of how the obstetric profession has been among the medical subspecialties least grounded in sound science. Additionally, such accounts were (and remain) useful in inspiring action: In response to emerging claims of questionable treatment by obstetric professionals, a small but vocal "free birth" movement formed in the midcentury United States, promoting the message that the antidote to unwelcome and unsafe obstetric care was to let nature take its course. After all, eons of human history verified that women had given birth successfully without extensive medical intrusion; returning to natural childbirth meant rejecting formal maternal medical care altogether, including hospital birth and professional obstetric care. Though the free birth movement failed to draw women away from hospital birth, its far-reaching effects can be seen among contemporary mothers planning a more natural birth experience.

STUDY MOTHERS EXPECTING NATURAL CHILDBIRTH

Twenty-five (33%) study mothers anticipated natural childbirth (vaginal delivery in or outside hospital, with other criteria varying by group, described in their respective chapters). Only 15 of those 25 are the focus of this chapter, for five mothers were pursuing natural birth outside hospitals and another five were planning vaginal birth after cesarean (VBAC), two unique circumstances that warrant separate treatment. This chapter's 15 women were demographically diverse, their education ranging from less than high school to graduate degrees and their income ranging from poverty level to affluent. Five (33%) had public insurance. Two mothers had neither a spouse nor a stable partner; the rest were married or partnered. Five (33%) were nonwhite or mixed race. Nine (60%) were primiparous (giving birth for the first time), and the rest were having second or third children. No mothers reported identified risk factors, though one mother was under significant psychosocial stress. Following the approach outlined in chapter 1, I discuss findings for the whole group with quotes and examples of experiences drawn from select representative cases; mothers' names are fictional.

In describing how they had arrived at their expectation of natural childbirth, three mothers spoke of the belief that childbirth was a natural function of the female body; in second-time mother Aisha's words, "Not to sound horribly sexist, being a woman and all, but our bodies were physically created to do this." Penny reflected on the potential of the childbirth function to empower mothers, describing her belief in "maternal empowerment" as a primary benefit. Focusing on fetal rather than maternal benefits, another four mothers mentioned pursuing natural childbirth based on their belief that the approach was best for their offspring; both Bella and Cherise specifically mentioned the benefits to newborns of birthing "without medication."

Mothers who had previously given birth related the effects of their previous experiences, both positive and negative, on their decisions. Aisha described an "amazing" first birth experience that inspired her to have a second intervention-free birth. Two experienced mothers said they anticipated repeating natural birth because their previous experiences had been, in Courtney's words, "wonderful." In contrast, Andrea described her natural birth decision as a reaction to a previous negative experience involving labor induction and an epidural she described as "awful" and as the "the worst thing you could do," largely because she found medication ineffective and an impediment to pushing.

Without the benefit of having yet given birth, all but one first-time mother spoke to the influence of others' advice and accounts as primary influences in their decisions for natural birth. For example, Penny had received an explicit message from her own mother: "She has made it abundantly clear … it's feasible to do that without an epidural or narcotics or anything … you get in there and you get it handled and you move on." Other first-time mothers took guidance from friends, either because they did not communicate well with their own mothers or because their mothers' experiences had been negative. Shelly said her own mother's births had involved extensive, "traumatic" medical intervention, as had her friends', leading her to consider natural childbirth for herself.

Jasmine had decided on medication-free childbirth in response to negative reports of epidural treatment from her own mother and positive accounts of hospital natural childbirth from friends. Heidi said others' reports only confirmed her intuition: "I actually never thought of anything else. Nothing ever had to convince me; … everything I read or people I talk to just assure me more." Two first-time mothers also mentioned pursuing natural childbirth partly based on fear of obstetric intervention, stated most clearly by Shelly, who said, "I'm more scared about the effects of epidural than I am of the pain of a vaginal delivery."

MATERNAL EXPECTATIONS FOR HOSPITAL NATURAL CHILDBIRTH

As can be seen in the chapter's opening quotes, contemporary mothers envisioned *natural childbirth* variously. However, one defining theme cut across all mothers' descriptions of their expectations for their own natural childbirth experiences: vaginal delivery. Correspondingly, nearly all mothers associated vaginal birth with the word *natural*; in one mother's expression, "it's a natural function." Though no mother in this group spoke to the expectation of greater maternal safety in vaginal birth than in cesarean birth—with the latter involving higher established rates of uterine rupture, aneurism, hemorrhage, and surgically induced infection (Clark et al., 2008; Hoyert, 2007; Kuklina et al., 2009; NIH, 2006)—two mothers framed vaginal birth as the mechanism for avoiding cesarean delivery, which to them signaled a medical emergency they wished to avoid.

All mothers in this group expected natural (as opposed to medically induced) labor onset. For example, first-time mother Shelly said, "She can come when she wants to come," and first-time mother Kayla used nearly the same words in describing her expectation of spontaneous labor. Two mothers in this group had had labor induced in previous births; one of those two anticipated avoiding the procedure this time, and second-time mother Andrea suspected but still hoped to avoid medical induction. Whereas all mothers anticipated spontaneous labor, two mothers dissented from the otherwise near unanimous, mildly negative view on labor induction. For example, one mother stated that she would undergo elective induction because "you just want to see them and hold them."

A third unifying theme emerging from this group's discussions of their childbirth expectations was to give birth without pain medication, particularly epidural analgesia. Though mothers expected not to avail themselves of medical pain relief, 100% of mothers anticipated childbirth pain, with first-time mother Jasmine saying, "I want to be able to share my story, even though it's painful." First-time mothers said they expected pain but "had no idea" about what to expect in terms of intensity, as Penny's statement shows: "I've read some women have such excruciating pain they'd rather be dead … some women orgasm during birth. I'm just hoping to be somewhere in the middle." By virtue of experience, multiparous mothers expressed their firsthand knowledge of the pain involved in childbirth, which Aisha described as "a horribly painful experience; there's just no covering that up."

Several mothers said previous experience had helped them prepare to use nonmedical pain-relief strategies: "I want to try all kinds of options that they give you and accessories like the ball and showers and bath … anything to distract my mind, I guess." In fact, nearly all mothers said they intended to employ some nonmedical pain-relief strategy, with five mentioning anticipated use of birth tubs or water, three mentioning doula support, and others mentioning individualized approaches such as birth hypnosis, relaxation strategies, or "keeping energy where you need to be" by "not screaming."

The fifth uniform theme among this group's mothers was to give birth without instrumental assistance (forceps or vacuum), but this expectation became clear only through prompting. In discussing their expectations of avoiding instrumental assistance, mothers made known a general objection to such procedures, and Shelly said, "I would hope that we wouldn't have to do the vacuum thing." Though mothers wanted to avoid instrumental assistance, they generally embraced fetal monitoring as, in one mother's words, "a good thing"; another mother commented, "You want to know how your baby is doing in labor." Along with those views, 100% of mothers in this group expected fetal monitoring; Bella, a first-time mother, was the only one who expected auscultation, and the others expected either EFM specifically or "whatever they do."

In response to prompting, mothers made apparent their uncertainty about whether to expect other hospital obstetric practices such as IV fluids, labor acceleration, or episiotomy—hesitation captured in one mother's statement that "I would not want to rush into that" and in another's reference to IAP, "If it has to be." Despite equivocation on whether to expect such obstetric intervention, mothers' views on those same procedures were generally mildly negative, shown in Cherise's statement that overall, she was seeking the least "medical experience … possible."

LESS FREQUENTLY MENTIONED EXPECTATIONS

Other childbirth expectations emerged within this subgroup but among fewer mothers. Thirteen mothers alluded to an expectation of having personal control over the birth situation, seen in Aisha's statement, "I pretty much run the show," and in Kayla's more elaborated view: "I should remain, for the most part, in control the whole time, and do what I want, and [make] the decisions."

Six (40%) mothers mentioned labor duration in their expectations, with third-time mother Courtney the only one to mention an expectation of long labor, reflecting her previous experiences with labors of over 30 hours. Three first-time mothers anticipated relatively short labors based on knowledge of their own mothers' experiences. Aisha said she expected her labor to proceed quite quickly: "When I say it's time to go, it's time to go, 'cause I go fast."

Seven (47%) mothers expected their pathways to result in good birth experiences. For two multiparous mothers, the expectation came from previous experience with supportive obstetricians; two others' expectations came from outside influences, such as the one mentioned by first-time mother Bella, who said, "I started reading stories of women who have done natural childbirth and that seemed to make a big difference in their birth." Other mothers framed the expectation of a good-quality birth experience in relation to those they had heard about. For example, first-time mother Shelly recalled that two of her close friends "regretted" their "traumatic" cesarean deliveries. Andrea said her own mother had accepted an epidural that she "wished she'd never gotten" and had been "anesthetized" in a later birth for reasons unclear to her, and Andrea expected to avoid both in her upcoming birth.

Perhaps reflecting the emphasis contemporary culture places on childbirth preparation and availability of resources facilitating this, only two first-time mothers mentioned not knowing what to expect. These statements did not come in the absence of any other expectation; for example, Bella reported an expectation of pain, but also said, "I don't know what to expect … so I guess I'll just freak out!"

Finally, eight (53%) mothers, of whom four were primiparous, described an expectation (and fear) of perineal tearing, which may occur in up to 85% of first-time mothers (Wheeler & Richter, 2007). As the fetus nears the vaginal opening, the perineum (tissue between the posterior vaginal opening and the anus) may not stretch sufficiently, especially when the fetus descends quickly, and the perineum may tear. Most cases are minor, grade I or II, treated by routine wound care or with stitches (DeFrances et al., 2007). Grade III or IV tears, or *perineal traumas*, involve vaginal muscles and the posterior wall (toward the anus); these tears occur in 0.3–9% of obstetric patients. Labor induction and other obstetric interventions place mothers at higher risk (Wheeler & Richter, 2007). Poor medical treatment is generally held to blame for perineal trauma in nations with advanced obstetric care (Berghella, Baxter, & Chauhan, 2008). Not surprisingly, perineal trauma places mothers at higher risk for intense negative emotions both immediately and in the longer term (Dudding, Vaizey, & Kamm, 2008). Mothers did not specify whether they anticipated minor or major tearing.

Greatest Fears in Childbirth

To elicit other expectations mothers might have not revealed upon direct questioning, I asked, "What is your greatest worry about your upcoming birth?" Most mothers mentioned more than one, but worry over newborn health, mentioned by eight (53%) mothers, ranked first. Four mothers mentioned childbirth pain as a chief concern, with Andrea stating her concern particularly strongly: "I'm worried if I'm in that kind of pain that I might start to lose it, and I'll get the epidural and it won't work again, and that would be the worst." Consistent with some first-time mothers' declaration of not knowing what to expect, three first-time mothers said they most feared "the unknown."

Other concerns appeared only once in individual mothers' reports, and included fear of labor induction (Andrea), fear of losing the baby (Bella), fear that her baby would not be a girl (Kayla), fear of becoming isolated postpartum (Heidi), and fear of losing control over personal behavior during labor (Shelly). Aisha worried that her obstetrician would not be available to attend her birth (he had notified her of vacation plans), in which case she said she would not go to the hospital.

Natural Childbirth Expectations Were Not Absolute

Although each mother expected and valued vaginal birth free of medical pain relief, labor induction, and operative assistance, not one said she would attempt to override a medical recommendation contrary to her expectations if fetal health were somehow at risk. For example, Bella said she would accept labor induction "if the baby was in danger." Of cesarean delivery, another mother said, "I'm not going to say, 'No, we're not going to do the c-section at all' … whatever is in the best interest of the baby is what I'm going for … if need be." And of any medical recommendation potentially violating her expectations, Cherise said, "If [the fetus is] in dire straits, then we'll do what has to happen."

Summary of Maternal Expectations for Hospital Natural Childbirth

Childbirth expectations shared among all mothers in this hospital-natural-childbirth group included expected vaginal birth, natural labor onset, expected pain addressed with various nonmedical strategies but not pain medication, no instrumental assistance, and fetal monitoring. Mothers had less certain expectations about receiving widely used obstetric interventions, such as internal monitoring and episiotomy, though their views on such procedures were generally negative. Some, though not all, mothers mentioned expectations related to control over childbirth-related decisions, labor duration, perineal tearing, having a good experience, and not knowing what to expect. It should be noted that no matter how many mothers held a particular childbirth expectation, no mother viewed hers as absolute; all women shared the view they would relinquish expectations if fetal well-being were at risk.

Based on the childbirth expectations all mothers in this group shared, it was possible to assess the relative match between expectations and experiences for the group as a whole, and those results are presented first. To provide a more complete image on the context of and the process by which mothers' expectations may have been confirmed or violated, it was necessary to examine individual cases, and representative examples are included. Following review of maternal responses to a question on satisfaction, I summarize and discuss results.

Confirmed and Violated Expectations in Planned Hospital Natural Childbirth

Of the 15 mothers who anticipated natural childbirth to include vaginal delivery, all reported childbirth pain and none reported instrumental assistance, consistent with their expectations. Six (40%) mothers' experiences met the full set of remaining expectations, including natural labor onset, no pain medication, fetal monitoring, and vaginal delivery; nine (60%) had one or more expectations violated. Three (20%) mothers had their birth mode violated by labored cesarean delivery, and two of these were first-time mothers. Seven (47%) had labor artificially induced with intravenous oxytocin. Seven (47%) mothers had pain medication; six received epidurals and one received systemic opiates.

Only two cases involved violation of a single expectation. Both these mothers received pain medication; one was administered systemic opiates and the other, an epidural. The remaining cases involved multiple violations. Of the seven mothers whose labor was artificially induced, six went on to have epidurals, continuing to anticipate vaginal delivery, and two of those went on to deliver by cesarean. One mother went into labor naturally but had an epidural and cesarean delivery. One mother whose labor was artificially induced could not use water to relieve pain as she had anticipated because of "required" internal monitoring.

CASES OF EXPECTANCY CONFIRMATION IN HOSPITAL NATURAL CHILDBIRTH

Most would agree that in childbirth, previous experience is a benefit, and Aisha's previous positive hospital natural childbirth with an obstetrician who she felt fully supported her needs led her to expect the same for this, her second birth. In fact, Aisha said things "went a little bit easier" and more quickly than she had expected. Within 45 minutes of realizing she had gone into labor, Aisha's partner took her from her home to the hospital. Upon arrival at the hospital, an unanticipated, much-welcome surprise greeted her: Her obstetrician had returned from his vacation to attend her birth. Aisha gave birth within two hours of being admitted; she reported, "It only took two pushes."

Speaking to the subjective definition of short labor, third-time mother Courtney described her lived birth experience as having confirmed and in some ways exceeded her expectations, partly owing to how "fast it happened this time." Her previous labors each having lasted over 30 hours, Courtney was pleasantly surprised at laboring for only 20 this time, spending 18 of those at home, during which time she and her husband "walked … probably about two hours, approximately three miles." Once in the hospital, Courtney said, she received IAP, which she had not expected but hardly noticed because "she came out really fast … I felt like I didn't have the stamina, I felt tired; I was afraid of the pain I knew pushing took … [but] overall, it was extremely quick."

Two mothers' childbirth accounts showed that previous births are not essential in arriving at experiences that closely match expectations. First-time mother Heidi, who said she felt "lucky" to have previously met and liked the midwife from her prenatal clinic who attended her birth, spent about three hours of her total five-hour labor in the hospital. She said childbirth for the most part aligned with her expectations, though she attributed the unanticipated intensity of her pain to rapidly progressing labor. Bella, another first-time mother, described her experience as "pretty similar" to her expectations, and of her total 12-hour labor (seven in hospital), she said,

> I kind of freaked out a little in the very beginning and had the thought of, 'Oh, now I kind of see why people ... rush to the hospital and want epidurals right away' ... And then I just totally calmed myself down ... though the actual pushing the baby out was more intense than I really could have even imagined.

These mothers' reports of labor duration evidence first the subjective and relative nature of the experience, with both Aisha and Courtney saying labor had progressed more quickly than they anticipated despite its lasting 3 hours for one and 20 for the other. On the other hand, no mother reported spending more than seven hours laboring in hospital; such duration presents no challenges to institutional and medical time lines for "normal labor." Still, labor duration conforming to medically defined limits of normality did not free any of these mothers from one or more unanticipated events stemming from routine institutional practice, and mothers responded to them in various ways.

For two mothers, those events arose during the childbirth process itself, beginning with Courtney's report of unanticipated IAP administration, which she apparently did not find too bothersome. For Heidi, who had anticipated EFM, the unanticipated experience came as a result of the process involved in obtaining EFM readings:

> They were so worried about the baby; they kept putting on heart monitors, they kept on saying, 'We're having trouble getting the baby's heartbeat, blah blah blah...' They were more worried about

> the baby … They kept … trying to measure stuff and monitor stuff … they totally ignored me even though I was right there in the center of everything.

She felt "out of the loop" with regard to her labor progress; Heidi was "shocked" at how quickly her fetus descended, and would have been considerably less distressed if staff had checked on her labor progress instead of continuing to attempt to obtain EFM readings. To her surprise, Heidi's newborn "came just after a few pushes," which left Heidi "really shocked and freaking out and traumatized," especially once staff started stitching up her extensive perineal tear. Overall, she said, she did not remember "much of it, it's all pretty much … a blur."

For both Bella and Aisha, unanticipated events came not in the birth process itself but after their newborns' arrivals. Bella's expressed fear of "losing the baby" was tested when an obstetrician appeared to accompany her midwife just as her newborn arrived, and staff immediately took her newborn out of the room to examine her. The next day, Bella said, "the midwife came in and said that if she'd been able to be alone or if the other midwife had been there, then that probably wouldn't have happened because she thought the doctor overreacted … The baby was fine."

Finally, consistent with her expectation of "running the show," Aisha requested hospital discharge "ASAP" after delivery, but her expectation was violated when staff reportedly told her she had to remain hospitalized for 48 hours. The first night, Aisha stayed on the obstetric ward; the second night, the ward was full, and she had to move to an adult acute care unit that she described as "awful."

Case of Single Expectancy Violation in Hospital Natural Childbirth

Saying she had come to "expect the unexpected" in childbirth, first-time mother Cherise did, however, anticipate in-hospital, medication-free vaginal delivery, and her expectations were met on two of those three counts. Anticipating a short labor like her own mother's, Cherise left for the hospital shortly after feeling intense contractions. After a few hours in the hospital's whirlpool with her doula and fiancé, Cherise said her labor stalled and her caregiver recommended systemic opiates to help her rest. She took the medication and "immediately went into transition," and her newborn arrived less than an hour later. Cherise described her obstetric caregivers, two midwives previously unknown to her, as "really warm," and she felt her care was "about taking care of me," and "making sure I was comfortable." She expressed no regrets about having received IV opiates during her total six-hour labor and said if she could go back and do anything differently, she would "honestly" not "change anything."

Cases of Multiple Expectancy Violations in Hospital Natural Childbirth

Reports from mothers whose experiences violated their expectations on multiple counts shared the feature of hospital labor that exceeded 12 hours. A negative tone characterized these accounts; most participants in this group attached positive language only to isolated aspects of the experience. In addition, each of these mothers' experiences confirmed one of the primary childbirth fears she had expressed during pregnancy. The seven of these eight mothers whose labor was induced as the first of the expectancy violations revealed a wish that labor had not been induced.

For three mothers, induction eventually led to expected vaginal delivery, but for each, additional expectancy violations crowded the labor and delivery pathway. Penny, who expected a natural childbirth pathway largely in response to her mother's strong opinion on the matter, had a nonstress test performed by her midwife about a week after her due date revealing "the amniotic fluid was kind of low." She recalled her midwife's saying, "As the amniotic fluid gets lower, it makes labor and delivery much more difficult," and she decided on labor induction after it was offered. Penny reported to the hospital the next morning and received IV oxytocin for induction; nine hours passed before she, exhausted by that point, accepted an epidural. Looking back, Penny said that had she "not been induced," she might have achieved the birth experience she had originally imagined, but "the Pitocin was just crazy to me ... which is why I didn't want to be induced in the first place."

Like Penny, second-time mother Andrea had hoped to avoid labor induction, citing a negative experience with it in her previous birth. After passing her due date by two weeks, Andrea met with her doctor, whose recommendation confirmed her earlier fear of having labor induced. She recalled her physician's saying, "'We are running late ... your placenta gets older, the baby gets bigger ... you just don't want to prolong it and have something happen.'" Saying his words "made sense" to her, Andrea accepted labor induction. She reported for induction the next morning; after laboring for about nine hours, her physician recommended an epidural on his suspicion that she'd be delivering "like a 10- or 11-pound baby." Andrea added, "I really wanted to fight for a natural birth, but [the obstetrician] said, 'You know, we may have to do a c-section' ... I was pushing for natural, but I didn't get to this time." Andrea delivered her 7 pound, 7 ounce baby about two hours later. Additional expectancy violations came later for Andrea, who returned to the hospital with her newborn shortly after discharge, where the baby was diagnosed with *E. coli*. Medical staff inquired whether her newborn had been around Iraq veterans or other hospitals; after an investigation, the hospital found that "the nurses and the people who were handling the baby weren't washing their hands."

Shelly's postinduction childbirth story became considerably more complex than either Penny's or Andrea's. About 11 days past her due date, Shelly underwent an ultrasound that indicated "amniotic fluid levels were low." For this reason, Shelly's doctor "felt that it was important ... to go ahead and be induced, and so they induced me." Shelly reported for labor induction, slept on and off overnight, and labored in a tub. But after staff struggled with external EFM, Shelly had to switch to internal monitoring, and her water labor was brought to a halt. After about 14 hours of laboring in bed, it seemed that Shelly's fear of losing control over personal behavior in labor was realized; she said, "I had what everyone kind of described as a psychotic break, I really just broke down ... I don't remember anything ... At the end of that, I was like, 'I'm done, give me an epidural.'"

Unfortunately, the anesthesiologist could not successfully place the epidural despite trying "seven times." Hours later, Shelly felt the urge to push, and her newborn arrived within six minutes, leaving Shelly with a grade IV perineal tear. Once things settled down, Shelly spent a few hours with her newborn, whom she described as "perfect," before things took another unfortunate turn. Her baby turned purple, was transferred to a high-level neonatal intensive care unit (NICU), and remained there for five days. Shelly's baby was eventually treated for an acute lung infection; Shelly said she was fine upon NICU discharge and remains so today. (Though rare, cases of serious neonatal infections secondary to internal fetal monitoring involving scalp incisions have been reported; see, for example, Freedman & Baltimore, 1990.) Looking back, Shelly said, "I would certainly prefer to not be induced. I mean I would really like to see what would have happened if my body had … gone into labor on its own."

Kayla and Jasmine, both first-time mothers, had their childbirth expectations violated by epidural administration and cesarean delivery; Kayla's journey down that road began with labor induction. She passed her due date by about a week and said her doctor wanted her to "go to the hospital to have labor induced." After being induced the next morning, Kayla labored for eight hours with little progress. She underwent amniotomy and then accepted an epidural offered by staff to "help her relax." Eleven hours later the analgesia had worn off, and Kayla felt exhausted:

> I just wanted her out of me. I had felt before like, oh, I don't want a c-section, but … I just wanted her out. So I asked like five times for a c-section, and after I'd asked for about the fifth time, the doctor came in and decided to do it.

Unlike Kayla, Jasmine went into labor naturally, and after laboring in hospital for a few hours, she said, "They thought she'd be a big baby … they wanted me to have some pain control … they gave me an epidural. I wasn't able to move." About eight hours later, the idea of cesarean delivery came about as a reaction to fetal status, Jasmine said. "Her heart rate was going up and down, up and down … they didn't want to stress the baby out anymore … He [the obstetrician] did tell me I could wait it out, but to not stress the baby out." Responding to her greatest worry of "a problem—like with the baby," expressed during pregnancy, Jasmine said she "went for a c-section," to avoid placing further stress on her fetus.

For both Kayla and Jasmine, surgery went smoothly. Like several other mothers, however, Kayla encountered additional unanticipated challenges while hospitalized. She believed medical staff misread her attempts to manage pain with relaxation strategies during labor—"just deep breathing … doing the things I'd read in books and seen on videos … just soothing myself"—as signs of psychiatric illness. Kayla said she had to convince the obstetric team that she was, in fact, psychiatrically stable. Her difficult birth and hospital experiences reinforced Kayla's conviction, which she had held (and disclosed to me) well before her newborn's arrival, that she would have no more than one child. Unfortunately, her physician's refusal to perform tubal ligation before discharge violated her earlier expressed personal expectation of having control over medical decisions and left Kayla saying, "I think, I'm 34; I know what I want."

SATISFACTION

All mothers in this group reported being satisfied or better; Heidi was the only exception, saying she "wasn't sure" whether she was satisfied. Of the mothers whose experiences confirmed expectations, Bella said she was overall "very satisfied," though she would have liked to stay home longer before going to the hospital. Heidi, Courtney, and Aisha all placed their statements of high satisfaction within the context of shorter than anticipated labor. Courtney and Aisha went further, saying they believed that their experiences had been made better by high-quality caregiving; Courtney described a particularly attentive nurse whom she remembered "doing a dance that she got to be part of a birth where they were going to announce what the baby was."

Mothers whose childbirth experiences violated expectations reported being overall satisfied, but each mother qualified her statement. For example, Shelly referred to the benefit of unmedicated birth for her newborn even though she "didn't enjoy" the experience "at all." Penny said she was "100% satisfied" with childbirth outside the fact that it violated her earlier and firmly held expectation of going medication-free, and instead involved medical labor induction in week 40 of pregnancy and an epidural in labor. Both Jasmine and Kayla said they felt "OK, satisfied," and as if seeking something to attach their satisfaction to, both women subsequently remarked on the better-than-expected appearance of their surgical scars. Jasmine said, "My scar looks like a scratch," and Kayla said, "He [the obstetrician] wasn't a butcher like everyone had said, [and] my scar was hardly visible."

Summary and Implications

Of this study's 15 mothers anticipating hospital natural childbirth with shared expectations of natural labor onset, no pain medication, fetal monitoring, and vaginal delivery, six (40%) achieved experiences consistent with that set of expectations. Within that group, however, one mother's personal expectation of control in medical decisions was violated by institutional requirements, and two other mothers had unanticipated experiences associated with aspects of medical care they found distressing. Nine (60%) mothers experienced a violation of one or more expectations among those applied to the whole group by labor induction, pain medication, internal fetal monitoring, cesarean birth, or a combination of those. The most frequent expectancy violation was the receipt of epidural analgesia, followed in frequency by artificial labor induction; cesarean delivery was experienced least often but affected 20% of women in this group.

In many ways, the match between mothers' expectations and experiences speak as much to technocratically oriented institutional expectations imposed on laboring women as they do to maternal views on childbirth before the fact. Medical expectations of "normal birth," which drive corresponding institutional practices (and vice versa) set firm standards for labor and delivery progress and duration (e.g., Zhang et al., 2010). Along those lines, mothers whose experiences (mostly) confirmed their personal expectations shared the feature of medically defined smooth and efficient labor that unfolded along an expected course and time line, beginning with natural labor onset near their predetermined due dates. These mothers' labor duration also met medical expectations, at least during hospitalization: Not one exceeded the seven hours Bella reported laboring in the hospital, and though Courtney's 20-hour labor would ordinarily push the limit of medically defined normalcy, spending 18 of those hours at home removed the opportunity for hospital staff to identify her time as deviant. With their bodies performing "on course," at least during hospitalization, minimal perceived need arose to address deviations with the obstetric interventions these naturally birthing mothers viewed as objectionable.

Institutional expectations also factored into the unanticipated (and unwelcome) events experienced by two mothers who otherwise had expectations confirmed. Heidi's report of repeated staff attempts to place an EFM belt reflected multiple aspects of contemporary, technocratically based institutional obstetric values: first, that ensuring fetal well-being should trump any maternal discomfort related to routine procedures such as EFM, and second—on a more practical level—that EFM is necessary and superior to the less intrusive (and in Heidi's case, perhaps easier to maneuver), old-fashioned auscultation option. Mandating a 48-hour stay for a mother like Aisha, who requested early hospital discharge, only to place her—an otherwise healthy person—on a ward with patients who had diagnosed illnesses reflects many of the contradictions operating within contemporary institutional obstetric care.

Further highlighting the technocratic paradigm by which contemporary obstetrics operates were accounts from mothers whose birth experiences did not conform to expected labor and delivery time lines, in particular, those seven mothers who had labor artificially induced. In each labor induction case, the mother described the decision-making process much like Penny and Andrea: A trusted obstetric caregiver raised a vaguely stated but non-life-threatening concern, such as low amniotic fluid or an aging placenta, followed by presentation of the "option" or recommendation to proceed with labor induction. In each case, mothers were left to accept or reject the proposed either/or remedy.

According to Kukla and colleagues (Kukla et al., 2009), childbirth is a momentous life event and therefore maternal childbirth decisions involve not only considerations of medical risk but also wider ranging concerns, such as the implications for one's personal birth narrative—reflected in Jasmine's expectation of being able to share her story, "even though it's painful." In communicating obstetric options surrounding important decisions (such as whether to induce labor), medical practitioners take the value-laden approach of presenting risks and benefits (as an aside, these mothers' reports lend the impression that only the risks of *not* inducing were presented), leaving mothers to decide largely on that basis alone. Not only does this numbers-based approach limited to medical risk leave mothers feeling abandoned (Kukla, 2005), it also positions them to behave as "moral pioneers" (C. Williams et al., 2005). Furthermore, this medical-numbers-only approach fails to take into account women's ability to make rational choices based not on medical risk alone but on a host of considerations important in their own lives (Kukla et al., 2009).

Given the generally negative tone woven throughout the accounts of this study's mothers who had anticipated natural birth but received labor induction, one of the many considerations accompanying optional or recommended labor induction would appear to be its potential influence on mothers' later memories and related accounts. In addition, mothers who had labor induced either directly expressed regret about having had the procedure or more mildly reported that they "wished" they had not received it. Finally, along with negativity and regret came another important story line: Labor induction triggered a chain of additional labor and delivery events that, one after another, violated maternal expectations. The chain of violated maternal expectations began when their labors (in all cases) exceeded standard institutional time lines, setting into motion standard obstetric responses—including amniotomy, epidural pain treatment, and higher than usual rates of cesarean delivery.

Of course, one could argue that mothers' expectations were violated because their birth processes were in fact deviant and thus expectancy violations were a necessary trade-off for ensuring their own and their offspring's safety and well-being. On that question, one can never truly know after the fact. It should be noted, however, that none of these seven mothers mentioned risk factors (one had high psychosocial stress) either before or after giving birth, other than passing their due dates and "low amniotic fluid." The 44% induction rate in this group, like the national induction rate in the United States in the 21st century, well exceeded the 10% rate recommended in the World Health Organization and the Pan American Health Organization's (1985) guidelines for scientifically and clinically sound labor and delivery care. Understandable as a mother's desire to conclude her pregnancy may be, no mother in this study had reached the 41-week mark for which labor induction has been shown to reduce risk of fetal death (Mozurkewich et al., 2009). In the present study, six mothers reported having had labor induced after passing their due dates by less than 11 days (estimated 39 weeks of pregnancy); the seventh, Andrea, was the latest, four days before week 41. Moreover, most mothers reported scheduling labor induction "just in case," creating a performance demand whose effects have not been systematically examined but should not go overlooked.

Taken as a whole, these mothers' accounts reveal the true rarity of a good match between naturally birthing mothers' expectations and experiences in hospital birth and the larger sphere of technocratically oriented obstetric care to which it belongs. Certainly, routines and procedures are a necessary component of running any large institution; without those, chaos would ensue. Perhaps refuge from a sense of *total* chaos brought about by childbirth's unknown factors partly motivates contemporary mothers anticipating natural birth to consider hospital birth even when they recognize the potential mismatch between their own and institutional orientations—knowledge reflected in Cherise's words, "I don't know if I trust the hospital's procedures," and in Bella's, "You don't necessarily need ten people hovering around you and hospital requirements, but the law cannot agree."

Maternal skepticism aside, it should be noted that regardless of whether mothers' childbirth expectations were confirmed, not one reported low satisfaction with the overall experience. In fact, the majority stated that they were satisfied or better. This finding seems inconsistent with much of the maternal narrative material contained herein, and speaks to the limitations of *satisfaction* as an adequate indicator of the mutually exclusive positive and negative events and emotional responses normally accompanying childbirth (Stolte, 1987). Relative maternal satisfaction in cases like these may instead be tied to larger, culturally based expectations of childbirth as something to be gotten through or survived more than welcomed and celebrated, with ultimate celebration attached to the arrival of a healthy newborn. In that case, whether maternal experiences meet expectations, particularly for mothers anticipating natural birth in hospitals, will rely primarily on physical factors and on dedicated caregivers like Aisha's doctor, who left his vacation to attend her birth.

Chapter 4

Expectations and Experiences of Planned Spinal (Epidural) Labor Analgesia

The Context of Contemporary Childbirth Pain Relief

In 2004, the American College of Obstetrics and Gynecologists (ACOG) and the American Society of Anesthesiologists (ASA) wrote, "There is no other circumstance where it is considered acceptable for an individual to experience untreated severe pain, amenable to safe intervention, while under a physician's care" (p. 213). Faced with its wide use in 21st-century childbirth—U.S. estimates range from 60% to 90%, depending on region and hospital (Osterman, 2009; Wong, 2009)—one might wonder why major medical organizations would take a stand on what seems self-evident: Dental patients readily accept medications to deaden the site of a tooth extraction, so why all the fuss over obstetric analgesia? Yet pain treatment in childbirth ranks among the most widely discussed if not controversial obstetric topics. A brief review lends some perspective on the sources of current concerns.

Analgesia refers to decreasing or altering the pain sensation, whereas *anesthesia* refers to blocking the pain sensation with or without loss of consciousness (Benzon, Raja, Molloy, Liu, & Fishman, 2004). In practice, labor analgesia should reduce childbirth pain but allow the mother to remain alert and move muscles to effect delivery. Anesthesia, on the other hand, effectively blocks pain but also blocks the transmission of nerve impulses necessary to move muscles, rendering the mother unable to push her newborn out (Benzon et al., 2004; Poole 2003). Childbirth analgesia originated more than 150 years ago with the use of ether and chloroform, powerful agents once used to anesthetize patients for surgery. In 1853, Britain's Queen Victoria began popularizing what she called "blessed chloroform" after her physician administered it during her eighth delivery (Pitcock & Clark, 1992). While obstetric anesthesia fast became wildly popular among British and U.S. mothers who could access it, opposition grew, initially from religious leaders who argued that childbirth pain was biblically scripted as penance for original sin (Cohen, 1996; Fulop-Miller, 1938). Nevertheless, scientists worked toward discovering safe and effective labor pain treatments, largely in response to maternal demand (Caton, 2009; Pitcock & Clark, 1992).

In the same early 20th-century decades that saw labor anesthesia increase in popularity, medical publications accumulated warnings of serious concerns, including maternal death and severe oxygen deprivation in newborns; mothers reported anesthesia's variable effectiveness, total loss of motor control, harsh physical restraint, and involuntary drug administration (e.g., Schultz, 1958). Such reports inspired concerned medical professionals and mothers to reconsider the merits of the so-called natural, or unmedicated, childbirth that women had historically endured. In 1944, British obstetrician Read published *Childbirth without Fear*, in which he proposed that labor pain had no true physiological basis, but that culturally constructed fear of the ensuing events caused muscle tension which in turn caused pain. The French obstetrician Lamaze similarly stated, "Painless childbirth is a fact" (1970,

p. 173), triggering the start of routine, hospital-based, prepared childbirth classes attended by thousands of 21st-century mothers in the United States each year.

Persuasive as "painless childbirth" arguments may have seemed at the time, researchers subsequently made clear that no matter how well prepared or relaxed a laboring mother might be, childbirth involves true physiological pain (e.g., Freedman & Ferguson, 1950; Melzack, 1984; 1993). Pain presumably originates from intense uterine contractions and cervical dilation, from pressure on organs and tissues during fetal descent, from stretching of the perineal tissues, and from the tearing of associated internal and external tissue. Childbirth also stresses the body, which in turn produces stress hormones associated with pain sensations (Benzon et al., 2004; Melzack, 1984; Wong, 2009). To natural childbirth advocates' credit, it is true that a psychological or affective component moderates pain. Pain receptors transmit messages to the brain, where those messages are translated in relation to, for example, one's past experience, perceived ability to endure pain, and sense of control over the pain (Dannenbring, Steven, & House, 1997; Melzack, 1993). In addition to increasing stress hormones, which in turn can intensify pain sensations, fear and apprehension can also lead to shallower breathing, making less oxygen available to the brain and to the organs and thus potentially influencing both pain perception and the birth process (R. P. Lederman, E. Lederman, Work, & McCann, 1985; Melzack, 1984).

For these reasons, contemporary natural childbirth techniques (generally) focus on shaping and managing pain perceptions rather than on instilling a belief that physical pain does not exist or that it can be eliminated. Although those strategies can be beneficial (e.g., Dannenbring et al., 1997; Simkin & Bolding, 2004), women on average report that childbirth pain exceeds that of phantom limb pain, cancer pain, or chronic low-back pain (Melzack, 1984). Despite evidence for the physiological basis of childbirth pain, controversies surrounding medical pain relief in childbirth continue, though they are apparently insufficient to trump the maternal desire for pharmacological solutions that motivated Queen Victoria 150 years ago to try a risky experimental procedure for reducing childbirth pain.

In the early 21st-century United States, epidural procedures are generally considered the professional (and maternal) medical pain-relief strategy of choice (ACOG & ASA, 2004; American Society of Anesthesiologists Task Force on Obstetric Anesthesia [ASATFOA], 2007). Administering one of its variants requires that the mother remain motionless during spinal injection(s) and placement of a catheter attached to an IV or pump for ongoing delivery throughout labor of medications similar to those used in dental procedures. An *epidural* involves a single injection (Nystedt, Edvardsson, & Willman, 2004; Poole, 2003) after which pain relief generally arrives in 15–20 minutes. A *combined spinal-epidural* (CSE) involves a second injection of a fast-acting opiate medication into the spinal fluid itself (University of Washington, 2010). Because CSE involves administering both a traditional anesthetic agent and an opiate, the anesthetic dose can be reduced, helping offset hypotension, which commonly occurs with epidural and can be worrisome; also, lower anesthetic drug doses allow for greater motor movement, earning CSE the nickname "walking epidural" (Collis, Davies, & Aveling, 1995; Rawal, van Zandert, Holmström, & Crowhurst, 1997).

Both epidural and CSE require obvious skill: Needles must be inserted at the correct site to ensure effectiveness, and incorrect placement can result limited or no analgesic effect, sometimes leading to repeat procedures. Properly placed, an epidural has been found to significantly reduce labor pain for about 90% of mothers (Melzack, 1993; Wong, 2009), though the extent of relief varies widely (Landau, 2009). In addition to lacking the desired effect in 10% of mothers, epidurals may cause infection at the puncture site (Simmons, Cyna, Dennis, & Hughes, 2007). The medications commonly cause nausea and vomiting. Anesthetic administration for more than six hours is associated with maternal fever (Anim-Soumah, Smyth, & Howell, 2005); maternal fever, in turn, has been associated with slightly higher rates of neonatal fever and adverse reactions to maternal fever treatment, leading to newborn assessment and admission to special care units (Segal, 2010).

Drops in maternal blood pressure are common and are usually treated with increased fluids, medications, or sometimes oxygen. About 1.5% of cases involve inadvertent piercing of one of the tough membranes closest to the spinal cord, causing headache or severe migraine (Wong, 2009). Though rare, bacterial meningitis cases have been reported, most likely related to poor sanitary practices or bacterial infection of the equipment or medication (Lurie, Feinstein, Hofetz, & Mamet, 1999; Roberts & Petts, 1990). Extremely rarely, anesthetic medication can travel to the mother's heart and stop it during labor, threatening the lives of both mother and neonate (University of Washington, 2010).

Epidural effects more commonly discussed include those affecting the labor process. Because it generally slows down the labor process, epidural administration has been associated with a higher probability of subsequent medical birth interventions, specifically, labor acceleration and instrumental delivery (Anim-Somuah et al., 2005; Simmons et al., 2007). Epidural administration has been associated with higher cesarean delivery rates, though not consistently; research on the matter is made difficult by the degree of cervical dilation at the time of analgesia administration, the specific procedures used, and the reason for administering the analgesia. One well-controlled study reported a 20% higher risk for operative delivery and 10% higher risk for cesarean delivery in primiparous mothers receiving epidural, and 14% higher risk for operative and 1.2% higher risk for cesarean delivery in multiparous mothers (Nguyen, Rothman, Demissie, Jackson, Lang, & Ecker, 2010).

Some 150 years ago, Queen Victoria popularized powerful and risky medical obstetric pain treatment, and since then, pharmacological means of minimizing or erasing labor pain have remained a chief maternal-care priority for both professionals and mothers. In the United States, the epidural has been widely promoted as the best available labor-pain treatment option, somewhat in contrast to a World Health Organization (WHO, 1985) recommendation that epidural be avoided as a routine treatment because of its associated risks to mothers and neonates. Though an exhaustive review of medical alternatives to the epidural is beyond the scope of this text, it should be noted that outside the

United States, other medical pain treatments are more frequently used in obstetrics. In particular, nitrous oxide (involving placing a mask over the mother's mouth and nose, often used in U.S. dentistry) is readily available on birthing units in other English-speaking nations and Scandinavia. Nitrous oxide allows the mother to control administration, and she can move freely, which is not possible with an epidural. Women report satisfactory pain relief with nitrous oxide, and it carries considerably fewer risks than does epidural analgesia (e.g., Rooks, 2007; Rosen, 2002). For all these reasons, the American College of Nurse Midwives (2009) issued a position statement recommending more widespread availability and use of nitrous oxide in obstetrics.

Despite concerns about the potential effects of epidural and about the availability of other options, epidural pain treatment appears to have become all but routine in U.S. hospital birth, performed on 60–90% of birthing women (Osterman, 2009; Wong, 2009). Complex and varied forces, some of them economic, likely figure into the epidural's dominance among obstetric pain treatments in the United States. To be direct, epidural administration generates hospital income. In addition, because an epidural can be performed only in a hospital, it limits mothers' choice of birth settings, drawing prospective center- or home-birth candidates in. Also in the mix, the professional assumption that women find the epidural most effective and desirable above all else limits both clinicians' and their patients' focus to the epidural as the single and best pain-treatment option. With that in mind, I turn to discussing women's expectations of and experiences with epidural pain treatment.

STUDY MOTHERS EXPECTING EPIDURAL

Twenty four (32%) mothers in this study reported a desire to have "epidural" or "spinal" pain treatment in childbirth, representing 39% of all mothers planning vaginal (as opposed to cesarean) birth. In addition to those 24 mothers, another 10 said they had considered epidural but that they preferred to defer their request until they had actually experienced labor pain. Distinguishing mothers planning from those deferring the epidural decision is the presence of labor stress: On the one hand, mothers planning a procedure in advance are, at least theoretically, making their decision in a less vulnerable state than mothers choosing to defer; a deferred request could be further complicated by staff input, labor progress, and anesthesiology staff availability. On the other hand, planning an epidural may reflect greater fear of childbirth and childbirth pain; fears are discussed in more detail later in this chapter. Given those factors distinguishing planned and deferred epidural decisions, I decided to treat these as two separate groups, with this chapter's focus on the 24 mothers who reported committing to a procedure in advance.

Mothers planning epidural varied in age (20 to 36 years), educational attainment, and income, with a few living at or below the poverty line and about an equal percentage reporting middle-to-high or high incomes. Three (13%) mothers were nonwhite. Two mothers were without spouses or stable partners. Twelve (50%) were primiparous. Eight multiparous mothers (75%) had received an epidural in a previous birth. No multiparous mother had delivered by cesarean, though four (25%) had previously had labor induced. Because of her history of serious kidney problems, one mother (Wendy) was identified as higher risk and saw a perinatologist for her care. Following the approach outlined in chapter 1, I here discuss findings for the whole group, citing quotes and examples of experiences drawn from select representative cases; mothers' names are fictional.

Mothers' reported reasons for planning epidural analgesia differed considerably between first- and later-time mothers. Seven first-time mothers reported that family members' and friends' accounts of positive experiences with epidural had influenced them to follow suit and schedule the procedure in advance. For example, Kelly's mother and several sisters had advised her to "get the epidural" based on their positive experiences with it. First-time mother Michelle was also following her own mother's path, saying she believed regional analgesia "would take care of any pain," her greatest childbirth concern. Abby's mother had gotten an epidural and had not spoken "negatively about the experience," so Abby had "firmly decided" to follow her mother's lead and her friends' advice. Valerie said that her mother had delivered several children at home and "didn't know about hospital birth," but her friends had advised her to "go for the epidural." In contrast, Luz made her decision to plan regional analgesia administration as a counter to her own mother's report of long and difficult medication-free labor.

Other first-time mothers referred to obstetric caregivers as influential in their decisions. For example, first-time mother Grace recounted that her obstetrician had suggested she consider a "spinal block." Wendy recalled her obstetrician's mentioning an epidural while educating her on how labor duration was "genetic"; aware that her own mother had labored "long, like about 23 hours," Wendy decided to plan an epidural.

Of mothers who had given birth before, nine (75%) had received an epidural in one or more of those births, and their previous experiences inspired them to plan the procedure again. Six of those mothers had not planned the procedure for previous births but decided this time to avoid laboring long in the hospital—Jen had labored for 10 hours and Noelle for 15 before receiving their respective epidurals. Of the three mothers who had planned epidurals in their previous births, Clare said she had made her interest known to all well in advance and had done the same this time around. The three mothers who had not previously had an epidural reported having wanted the procedure but being unable to receive it because they had arrived at the hospital "too late."

EXPECTATIONS OF MOTHERS PLANNING EPIDURAL

Like naturally birthing mothers, 100% of mothers in this group expected vaginal delivery. Views on cesarean delivery were negative across the board, evidenced in statements such as "It's hard on your body and you have to worry about your baby," and "Scary—cutting into muscle ... doesn't seem like the easy way out." In addition to expecting vaginal delivery, 100% of these mothers expected an epidural procedure to be part of their childbirth experience. Most mothers used the term *epidural* in reference to the procedure they anticipated, with one exception. First-time mother Grace initially said she had "decided against an epidural" but would have, upon her physician's recommendation, a "spinal block," which she described thus: "Unlike an epidural, it addresses pain in the pelvic region but allows mother to get up and move around and control pushing better." The procedure she described was most likely CSE (see the preceding discussion of spinal analgesia procedures).

Nineteen (79%) mothers reported having notified their obstetric providers of their wishes, whereas the remaining five mothers said they intended to do so in an upcoming prenatal visit. The interview itself may have influenced one mother's decision. When asked about what she expected to happen in childbirth, first-time mother Valerie initially said she expected to "have it all happen naturally, no epidural," as her mother had done in multiple home births. After saying "pain" was her greatest worry about childbirth, however, Valerie recalled that her friend had recently told her about a good experience with an epidural; then Valerie said she was "open to epidural" and intended to let her obstetric caregiver know at her next prenatal visit.

Without prompting, 20 mothers in this group explicitly expressed the expectation that childbirth would be considerably more manageable with an epidural. Framing that expectation most directly, first-time mother Iris said she expected labor and delivery to be "easy," adding, "Epidural, and I'm fine." Clare, pregnant with her third child, reported that her two previous labors had gone easily and without complications, and she attributed her relative success to the epidural.

With experience as their guide, the nine multiparous mothers who had previously had epidurals expected a repeat analgesia experience as good as or better than earlier ones. Three had planned epidurals in previous births; Clare said that she would not consider forgoing the procedure because "I have almost 10-pound kids, and they're just big; I tear." Six mothers had deferred their epidural decisions in previous births but decided to plan this time, and they expected that planning would result in more timely receipt of an epidural than had occurred in their previous births. For example, second-time mother Sarah had accepted an epidural after hospital labor of about 15 hours and, believing it "makes everything happier," had planned the procedure this time.

Six of 20 total mothers expecting an epidural to lead to a more manageable experience also expected the procedure to provide some, but not complete, pain relief; five of these mothers were giving birth for the first time. Wendy, for instance, expected some pain with labor onset, saying, "Everybody says that it hurts really bad ... I'm just waiting to figure out what happens." Along similar lines, first-time mother Luz expected "some pain and discomfort" but believed analgesia would "help with a lot of that." Though she had given birth once before, Sarah anticipated entering the unknown territory of natural labor onset, expecting a "different sort" of pain than what she had experienced with labor induction accompanied by an epidural she found effective.

In addition to expecting epidurals, mothers in this group expected some form of fetal monitoring, and most expected IV fluid administration. One mother, whose previous labor had been induced after she went postdate and had "low amniotic fluid," had scheduled labor induction to avoid repeating the "risk of going overdue" but anticipated natural labor onset before that time. No mother mentioned an expectation of having her own status monitored in childbirth. No mother expected labor induction. Though two mothers had previously had labor induced and hoped to avoid it this time, views on the procedure reflected a general sense that induction is warranted within a week or so of passing one's due date: "It's not good for them to ... cook too long"; "I wouldn't want the baby to be at risk in some way ... in there too long and getting too big, and not developing properly; also I would probably be quite uncomfortable." Mothers did not generally expect labor acceleration, systemic analgesia (with one exception), episiotomy, or instrumental assistance. Again, maternal views indicated a general acceptance of such procedures, reflected in the oft-repeated phrase "If you need it." No mother in this group explicitly mentioned expecting to use nonmedical pain-relief strategies.

EXPECTATIONS MENTIONED LESS FREQUENTLY

Eight of this group's 12 first-time mothers (75%) spoke of expecting a good childbirth experience in relationship to reports of family and friends; most had heard positive accounts that led them to hold similarly positive expectations of the epidural and the overall birth experience. Two of the four mothers who had not received epidural analgesia in previous births explicitly stated the expectation that planned epidural would lead to an experience better than a previous unmedicated birth. For example, in response to her previous unmedicated birth, which she described as "frantic," Jen said this time around she expected pain medication to allow her to "enjoy being at the hospital before I have … a midwife or a doctor really do their job … I don't want it to be an emergency situation—I want it to not be as frantic, I guess." Khala, who had previously given birth in hospitals in her native country overseas, said she looked forward to having an epidural, which had not been available on obstetric wards in her home country.

Three mothers mentioned their expectations of specific labor duration. First-time mother Wendy anticipated a long labor like her own mother's. Second-time mother Fae expected her upcoming labor to be shorter than her first. Second-time mother Jen anticipated a short labor, and aware that she might not arrive at the hospital in time for epidural administration, she said, "I'd be disappointed if I didn't get what I wanted."

Three first-time mothers said they were uncertain about what to expect, as in Marissa's statement, "I've read and gone to classes, but how can you really know?" Additional expectations were mentioned by only one mother each, and included one first-time mother's expectation of "panic" during labor (Alana); first-time mother Grace expected to be able to move about and find a comfortable position following the "light dose" of analgesia her physician had discussed, and one mother (Alana) anticipated the "excitement of meeting the baby."

Greatest Fears in Childbirth

To elicit other expectations mothers might have not revealed upon direct questioning, I asked, "What is your greatest worry about your upcoming birth?" Though six mothers did mention an expectation of childbirth pain, only one (Grace) mentioned pain as her top worry. Instead, the majority of mothers in this group worried chiefly about their newborns' well-being, with 19 (75%) explicitly expressing concern similar to Wendy's about "something happen[ing] to my baby" or similar to Sarah's worry that "the baby wouldn't be 100% healthy when [it] came out." Clare focused on possible occurrences within the delivery process itself, worrying that, "something will happen … that causes the baby to have any kind of harm … problems like shoulders getting stuck or cords wrapping around." Four mothers (17%) cast their concerns about labor and delivery more broadly, reflected in Luz's worries about "any unforeseen complications." Two mothers (Noelle and Luz) worried about the possibility of a labored or emergency cesarean delivery.

Worry that they would arrive at the hospital "too late" for epidural administration preoccupied one first-time and two later-time mothers. First-time mother Michelle put the matter simply: "If I don't get to the hospital in time, [I don't] get the epidural." With previous short labors as her guide, Clare echoed that worry, saying she hoped to get to the hospital as quickly as possible once in labor to get an epidural "just because I go so fast."

Concerns about arriving at the hospital too late for epidural administration beg clarification. Studies have shown that fast-acting epidural analgesia can be safely administered in advanced labor up until the point at which the baby has crowned (Pace et al., 2004). However, specialized anesthesiology staff must be readily available, particularly in quickly progressing, advanced labor. The mother must also remain still, which can be challenging in labor's final hours.

SUMMARY OF EXPECTATIONS IN MOTHERS PLANNING EPIDURAL

Like their naturally birthing counterparts, 100% of mothers planning epidural anticipated vaginal delivery, and two mothers reported labored or emergency cesarean as among their childbirth fears. Most of this group's mothers expected the epidural to make childbirth overall more manageable, basing their expectations on others' reports or their own experiences; along those lines, no mother reported any expectation or concern that an epidural might be ineffective. Fewer mothers expressed expecting pain at some point in the labor process. Although no one reported expectations of maternal monitoring, 100% did expect fetal monitoring. Mothers did not generally expect other widely practiced obstetric procedures, such as labor induction, labor acceleration, or episiotomy, but their reports indicated openness to them.

Mentioned less frequently were maternal expectations of having a birth experience better than a previously unmedicated birth and excitement about meeting the newborn. Two mothers expected labor of a specific duration; one of these mothers anticipated short labor and worried, as did two others, about getting to the hospital in time for administration. Worries about newborn health topped mothers' childbirth concerns, though no one explicitly stated a more specific concern related to possible negative effects of epidural on the newborn. Also absent from any mother's reported expectations or fears was reference to possible undesirable or negative effects of epidural procedures on her own well-being.

Confirmed and Violated Expectations in Epidural

The two defining childbirth expectations of mothers in this group were vaginal birth and receipt of epidural. Under those criteria, 14 (59%) of this group's 24 mothers had childbirth experiences that met those two expectations. However, nine of those, constituting the majority of women whose expectations were generally confirmed, experienced unanticipated childbirth events that had not figured into their earlier expressed expectations. Of the remaining 10 (41%) mothers, who had a major expectation violated, seven experienced a single violation involving either not receiving analgesia or perceiving the procedure as ineffective. Multiple violations occurred for three (13%) mothers for whom cesarean delivery constituted one of those violations. Ten (41%) mothers had labor induced.

Cases of Expectancy Confirmation

The five mothers whose childbirth expectations of receiving epidural pain treatment and delivering vaginally were confirmed without some other unanticipated event shared the common experience of laboring for less than five hours in the hospital. For example, of the two mothers who experienced natural labor onset, multiparous mother Noelle had previously had labor induced and was glad that this time labor began naturally shortly after her water had broken. Her newborn arrived about three hours later. Noelle said, "I had never experienced my water breaking on its own; I had never experienced contractions starting on their own … it was actually better than having an induced labor." Because things progressed so quickly, Noelle added, "They almost didn't have time to place an epidural … I could have done without it." Given her generally positive view on natural as opposed to induced labor onset and her apparently smoothly progressing labor, one has to wonder whether unbearable pain or difficulty shifting from an earlier firm decision to have an epidural led Noelle to go ahead with the procedure.

Third-time mother Clare, who had worried during pregnancy that she might not arrive at the hospital in time to get an epidural, had also worried about large fetal size because she'd already delivered two babies over 10 pounds. Therefore, Clare was not surprised to have her third labor induced about a week before her due date, as her first two had been. Clare attributed her total five-hour, "calm and peaceful and superfast" labor not to any specific medical procedure but to having a "great doctor" whom she had known for several years and to having exercised regularly throughout pregnancy. Like Clare, second-time mother Jen had no firm opposition to labor induction, so having labor induced after her water broke did not perturb her. From "the time they induced" after her arrival at the hospital, Jen said, labor lasted about five hours, and she described her experience overall as "easy; it was quick, and it was painless … I didn't feel anything."

Cases of Expectancy Confirmation with Unanticipated Events

Other mothers reported having achieved vaginal birth and receiving epidural pain treatment as they had expected, but unanticipated events arose as the labor and delivery process unfolded. All nine cases involved labor induction followed by epidural administration, with the mothers' descriptions of subsequent birth events reflecting one birth intervention's triggering the use of another in the cascade effect. For example, first-time mother Luz, who during pregnancy said she would readily accept labor induction "if necessary," passed her due date by a week and her "doctor decided that they wanted to induce by the 41st week … it seemed like the right decision, since we'd been waiting a while already." Expecting that induction would set labor and delivery on a "very … by the book" course, Luz found herself surprised by some of the twists and turns and cascading interventions in her 10-hour labor, including amniotomy, stopping and starting oxytocin alongside her fetus's heart-rate fluctuations, receiving "saline in the womb," then more oxytocin, and, to her surprise, her doctor's "deciding" to perform an episiotomy.

First-time mother Michelle, whose top childbirth fear had been getting to the hospital in time for epidural administration, also reported a labor experience that began with induction and was characterized by a subsequent cascade of interventions to control her labor's course. After Michelle had passed her due date by a few days, her physician scheduled induction for nine days later. Well before then, however, Michelle started having contractions and went to the hospital "because the pain was too much … it was too unbearable to stay at home." Because she was not dilating, hospital staff "had to do it. You know, the Pitocin drip, and break my water for me … all of that … the epidural …happened very fast, so I liked that." Her obstetrician increased and decreased oxytocin to balance a concern to keep Michelle's "contractions moving along" with concerns about fluctuating fetal heart rate. Nine hours later, Michelle's baby arrived.

Two experienced mothers who had hoped for (though not expected) natural labor onset also had labor induced and, as with both Luz and Michelle, attempts to control the labor's course involved stops and starts in multiple procedures and medical directives along the pathway to delivery. Sarah's labor was induced seven days before her due date because she "had low fluid at times." Having had a previous straightforward induced labor experience, Sarah was surprised by reports of fetal heart-rate fluctuations and subsequent oxygen administration and a directive against pushing because her fetus's heart rate had "bottomed out because … her cord was tied around her neck … and I had to stop for a couple of hours.” While she was waiting for the green light to push, Sarah’s analgesia wore off, and when she requested more medication, her physician cautioned her that it could lead to cesarean birth, so she decided against it. Of the total seven hours she spent in labor, Sarah said, “It was kind of a bummer … two hours without any medicine … once they let me push, I think she was out in like two minutes … it was no big deal after they finally let me push.”

Two mothers’ labor and delivery experiences confirmed or exceeded expectations, but unanticipated events occurred with their newborns. For Iris, a first-time mother whose quote “Epidural, and I’m fine” reflected the faith she placed in the procedure to help her through childbirth, the labor and delivery experience went much as she had anticipated. A day before her due date, Iris’s water broke and she reported to the hospital. As labor became more painful, she requested an epidural before “the point that I was miserable … I told them I wanted it …they gave it to me … from then on I was just happy.” Of her 18 hours of labor, 12 of which were spent in the hospital, Iris said, “It was just sort of casual … like they show on TV … we were just talking and pushing … really easy and no problem—piece of cake.” As easily as Iris’s labor went, her greatest fear of a newborn complication was tested. Concerns over possible newborn infection led medical staff to place Iris’s baby in the “little nursery” shortly after birth:

> They just wanted him to be on an antibiotic, and so they made it seem like he was so sick … since we’ve brought him home, no problems … I think it was just precautionary … I was sure he was going to die, but I don’t think that anything was really wrong.

Khala, who had previously given birth in a country where obstetric epidural was unavailable, described her experience as “total wonder; it was bliss.” Her eight-hour labor, about five hours of which occurred in the hospital, proceeded straightforwardly. Khala said,

> I was excited … absolutely no pain … everything they predicted happened … a lot of support from the doctors and the nurses, they

> were absolutely amazing ... they spoke to me like a friend ... they chatted ... they didn't dictate what was supposed to happen ... I had absolutely nothing to fear because ... I listened to them; it was spot on.

Khala's total eight-hour labor proceeded almost problem free until her fetus's shoulder became lodged in the birth canal and broke. (At least one study has shown higher risk of birth trauma associated with epidural administration; Perlow et al., 1996.) After letting Khala meet her newborn, staff took the baby to neonatal intensive care, where she stayed for three days. Khala said she and her baby are doing "wonderfully" today.

Cases of Single Expectancy Violation: Not Receiving Epidural

Five (21%) mothers did not receive an epidural as they had anticipated because either no anesthesiologist was available or they were told labor was too far advanced for analgesia administration. None of these mothers had earlier expressed an expectation that analgesia might be unavailable owing to advanced labor or any other reason. However, the hopes that Valerie and Grace held for short, uncomplicated labors like their own mothers' hinted at what lay over the horizon for them.

One day before her due date, first-time mother Valerie felt mild contractions, her water broke, and she went into "hard, active labor." She quickly reported to the hospital and requested "an epidural," and Valerie said staff told her, "'You're too far along; you can't have it.'" So she "just elected not to have any medicines ... did it natural." Valerie spent under three hours in the hospital before her baby arrived. Like Valerie, Grace's labor was in the three-hour range (3.5 hours, to be precise), but she labeled it "complicated" because "it was so fast." With labor progressing as quickly as it did, Grace was not able to have the epidural procedure she had anticipated because

> there wasn't time. It was so fast ... I thought I would be doing all these different positions and things during the labor ... I didn't want to labor on the bed ... my labor didn't go like that ... They said they needed 20 minutes of fetal monitoring, and then she was

> born. By the time the anesthesiologist was there … I was ready to push … It took her a while to get to the hospital.

Nevertheless, Grace found labor painful and recalled screaming and hearing her physician say to her, "You need to be quiet." Overall, she felt relieved that she had not used pain medication in labor, believing it resulted in a baby who "came out so perfect … she wasn't mashed up from forceps … she had great color … a 10 on the Apgar."

Cases of Single Expectancy Violation: Ineffective Pain Relief

Three (13%) mothers reported that in one way or another, epidural analgesia failed to live up to the expectations they had reported during pregnancy of complete or effective pain relief. In first-time mother Alana's case, epidural analgesia wore off during the 25 hours of her 30-hour labor spent in the hospital, with IAP adding to her pain:

> [IAP] honestly hurt me more than anything else … acid in my veins … Each nurse would think, oh, we need to bump it up a notch … I'd be literally crying, not knowing what to do from the pain, in a panic … I got burned and burned and burned over and over again.

After her first epidural dose wore off, Alana requested additional medication, but her nurse refused, saying the fetus must have blocked the analgesia's effects. An hour later, the anesthesiologist appeared and increased Alana's medication, which had "completely worn off" by the time the attending obstetrician "brought the mirror so I could see his [the baby's] head, and that really helped me sort of keep pressing on … the next thing I knew … I rocketed that big old head out of there!"

Like Alana, Fae found that her epidural provided much less relief than she had anticipated. She had labor induced just as she had done with her firstborn and for the same reason: "low amniotic fluid." With her labor progressing rapidly, she said her analgesia did not have time to "kick in" over the course of her six-hour labor. Shortly after her newborn's arrival, unanticipated adverse analgesia consequences set in:

> They inadvertently gave me a spinal tap ... the aftermath of the epidural and spinal tap was pretty bad ... severe headaches, back, and neck pains. Then they had go in and give me another epidural for seizures; it's called a blood patch, [and] it's to counteract the after symptoms ... Then after we got home I had to go back into the hospital to get another procedure because the first one didn't work. It was horrible.

Cases of Multiple Expectancy Violations

Three mothers' expectations of vaginal birth were violated with labored cesarean delivery. For first-time mother Marissa, expectancy violations included unsatisfactory pain reduction with the epidural and cesarean birth. Marissa's labor started on her due date, and she spent 12 hours at home before reporting to the hospital, where she received an epidural right away. Labor initially proceeded quickly, but "he didn't want to come out." An obstetrician entered her room, and Marissa said he offered to perform a cesarean before or after his upcoming break. She pressed on but during this time, Marissa said, her labor and delivery nurse repeatedly advised her to "go for the c-section" to avoid having to "get it all rebuilt down there." Marissa had cesarean surgery about two hours later, saying she felt everything, "like a fish flopping on the table ... every cut and stitch. I couldn't breathe it was so horrible, and they said I had to get through it because they couldn't give me anything else." Marissa took solace in the procedure's relative brevity compared to her 13-hour hospital labor, but she wondered whether the epidural had led to the need for cesarean.

For first-time mother Wendy, at higher risk because of a history of kidney problems, childbirth not only tested her expectations and her fears but also sounded life threatening and traumatic. After diagnosing her with preeclampsia, Wendy's obstetrician induced labor as soon as amniocentesis results indicated that delivery would be safe for her fetus.

Preeclampsia medications interfered with induction, however, so labor progressed slowly. She got an epidural and "I wouldn't dilate … on the third day he was all, 'We're gonna … deliver you in the morning…' There was nothing I could do … they just told me that I had to do it." Wendy could not recall much about the surgery, but after she was taken to recovery, things took a bad turn. She hemorrhaged, contracted high fever, and required a blood transfusion. She said, "The doctors told me I almost didn't make it … I was in there [the hospital] a week after I had the transfusion 'cause I was still having fevers… They didn't know why, and they still don't know why." Unfortunately, Wendy's baby also struggled, with repeat hospitalizations in her first weeks of life for "breathing problems and fevers" of no reported known origin. Wendy said her and her baby's health had improved somewhat.

SATISFACTION

With a few exceptions, mothers in this group reported being satisfied or better with their overall childbirth experiences, and mothers whose experiences confirmed their expectations and involved no unanticipated events discussed their outcomes most unequivocally. For example, Noelle and Clare reported being "very satisfied," and Clare used the term "100% satisfied." Mothers whose experiences confirmed expectations but involved an unanticipated event surrounding fetal or newborn well-being reported similarly unqualified satisfaction; for example, Khala said, "The easy way isn't necessarily the bad way, like what we were taught … to take pain relief really, really makes a big difference, and it makes it more enjoyable … you mustn't be afraid."

It is worth noting that each of these mothers, like others whose expectations were generally confirmed, attributed her overall positive views on childbirth to factors either in addition to or unrelated to the epidural she received. For example, Noelle experienced spontaneous labor as "better than" her previously induced labor and declared that she "could have done without" an epidural over the course of her five-hour labor; Noelle's report of being "very satisfied" with childbirth could have easily related as much to the smooth unfolding of the birth process as to any medical procedure she underwent. Clare's report of having been cared for by a "great doctor" she had known for years and Khala's report of obstetric staff who were supportive and "absolutely amazing" both lent the impression that their satisfaction arose as much from caring staff as from any specific procedure. Further confirming that maternal views on specific procedures are closely connected with the manner in which staff administer them and the way they treat mothers more generally, Michelle, whose childbirth expectations were basically confirmed, qualified her report of being "pretty satisfied" with reference to her postpartum care. "I thought they would be more attentive … I had heard through the parenting classes that they would come around and give you a sitz bath … I was there for days and nobody did anything like that."

On the other hand, women who either did not receive the epidural they had anticipated or who experienced negative epidural effects singled out the procedure in discussing their satisfaction levels. Among mothers whose expectations of epidural were violated either by ineffectiveness or by not having received it, Grace said she was so satisfied with her unmedicated birth that she couldn't "wait to have another kid," recalling her labor and delivery as "perfect." Even so, Grace said, she would prefer to have arrived at the hospital in time for epidural administration. Given Grace's description of her birth experience as "perfect," one has to wonder whether her continued interest in having an epidural related to the rosy picture her physician painted of the procedure for her during pregnancy or to lingering feelings she might have had about her physician's reported directive to "be quiet" when she screamed in pain during her otherwise uncomplicated and short labor. Like Grace, Valerie reported being "very satisfied" with her unmedicated birth but continued to wonder about the epidural she had not received: "I would rather have an epidural … [The pain was] a lot more intense than I thought it would be … I'm still undecided about it." Having received advice from a close friend to have an epidural, having set her mind on it beforehand, and having been denied the procedure she expected once she arrived at the hospital, Valerie was equivocal about her experience. Her hesitation is somewhat less surprising than Grace's. Not at all surprising was Fae's statement that her birth experience would have been considerably better "without the epidural nightmare" caused by inadvertent membrane puncture during epidural placement and the resulting migraine, rehospitalization, and additional spinal procedures. As if to convince herself that something bad was bound to happen in childbirth, Fae commented, "There's always something; nothing is ever perfect."

Perhaps resigned to her experience, which strayed far from expectations, Marissa said she felt "OK" about how labor and delivery unfolded for her. However, she said she "didn't want to think about it too much," feeling that much of what happened had been out of her hands. Similarly, Wendy attributed her complicated birth experience to having been "so sick," and in reference to the joy she felt with her newborn, she said she would easily repeat the experience if she could do so in good health.

From this entire group of mothers, Alana emerged as the only one who made a clear statement of dissatisfaction, saying she "didn't get to have the birthing experience" she had wanted and that she believed she "deserved a better experience with the epidural." Neither Fae nor Alana, whose epidural experiences went badly, said she would forgo an epidural if she could do it over again; instead, both women focused on a wish that the procedure had gone better than it did. In Fae's terms, that would have meant having her medical team "do the epidural correctly," and for Alana, it would have meant taking a stronger self-advocacy stance: "[I'd be] much more vocal about my pain medication ... when it's wearing off, they need to get someone in ASAP ... if you can't give me more epidural, then what else have you got?"

SUMMARY AND IMPLICATIONS

Cross-cultural evidence, scientific studies, and direct maternal reports have established that childbirth pain is, in fact, real and universal, and the 21st-century obstetric pain treatment of choice in the United States is the obstetric epidural. Twenty-four (39%) of this study's mothers planning vaginal birth decided well before going into labor that they wished to take advantage of what is widely presumed the best available option, and all who expected to undergo the procedure anticipated that it would help make childbirth better overall. Mothers apparently remained committed to the procedure for the remainder of pregnancy and into childbirth itself, for none reported requesting at any point that they not receive an epidural.

Advance planning of epidural pain treatment reflects an acceptance of a technocratic model of birth, a perspective further reinforced by these mothers' general acceptance of—though not necessarily expectations of having—other technological birth interventions (e.g., labor induction, acceleration, EFM). Among these mothers with a more technocratically oriented view on birth, 14 of 24 had their two-pronged vaginal delivery with epidural expectations confirmed. That number translates into a 59% expectancy-confirmation rate, outstripping less technocratically oriented, natural hospital-birthing mothers' 38% expectancy-confirmation rate by a full 21 percentage points.

However, expectancy confirmation in this group did not equate to the absence of any unanticipated events, for 9 of 14 mothers—well over half—whose original expectations of vaginal birth with epidural were sent awry by, for example, an aggressively managed yet unexpectedly (at least from mothers' perspective) variable labor and delivery course. A mother's decision to plan an epidural marks greater receptiveness toward obstetric intervention, which in turn likely resulted in the apparent lack of negativity or low negativity about having received unanticipated procedures. For example, consistent with national statistics, for 10 (41%) mothers in this group, labor was artificially induced, eight reportedly because of "low amniotic fluid." None of these mothers expressed regret about having undergone induction. In fact, though no mother directly expressed this view, labor induction might have assuaged concern about if or when pain relief would arrive because having labor medically initiated in the hospital practically guarantees timely epidural administration. Maternal openness to or perhaps trust that technologically advanced care operates in the offspring's best interest appeared to have translated into two mothers' relative lack of negative responses to their newborns' NICU hospitalization postpartum (though time's passage may have had some ameliorative effect).

Further underscoring the critical importance mothers placed on technologically advanced pain relief were qualities apparent within maternal accounts of unavailable or ineffective epidural analgesia, seen in 33% of this group's total cases and constituting the majority of expectancy violations. Despite stating the clear belief that unmedicated birth was better for their newborns, mothers' postpartum statements of lingering desire or ambivalence about not having received expected epidural treatment revealed an ongoing conviction that an epidural might have led to a better overall birth experience, even better than the "perfect" experience Grace described. Among mothers for whom epidural was ineffective or only partially effective, none stated regret over having had the procedure, only that they wished it had gone better. This lack of regret seemed particularly striking in Fae's report of an "epidural nightmare" involving accidental spinal tap, repeat spinal procedures, and repeat hospitalization.

Mothers who, like Fae, experienced a single expectancy violation were separated from those with multiple violations and subsequently more complicated labor-to-delivery pathways by their hospital labor times of 12 hours or less. In addition to laboring more than 13 hours in the hospital, mothers with multiple expectancy violations also underwent cesarean delivery, violating this group's across-the-board expectation of vaginal birth. Even with their relatively more open attitudes toward technocratic birth than their hospital natural-birth counterparts, this study's mothers who anticipated epidural drew the line of personally acceptable obstetric intervention at cesarean delivery.

Previous studies have shown that labored cesarean delivery is associated with more negative views on the birth experience (e.g., Carter, Frampton, & Mulder, 2006; Olde, van der Hart, Kleber, & van Son, 2006), evidenced in part here by Marissa's expressed preference to avoid discussing her childbirth experience. As much as cesarean birth may violate a mother's expectations, attributing the whole of her lingering distress to the delivery mode itself may be inaccurate; the role of professional expectations and related communication on mothers' receipt of the procedure are worthy of some attention. Specifically, by both Marissa's and Wendy's reports, medical professionals appeared to have decided to perform surgery before communicating with them, and Marissa's physician attempted to give her some control in the decision by offering a choice in the timing of the surgery. Also by their own reports, neither mother's situation was so urgent as to warrant true emergency cesarean delivery involving on-the-spot general anesthesia and surgery. Upon my prompting, neither mother described having been offered any alternative to cesarean delivery, such as instrumental birth, reflecting a medical perspective focused only on the surgical option, thus limiting mothers' associated views on their options and their sense of control over them.

Although planning an epidural reflects an overall orientation toward technocratic birth, it also reflects a mother's exercise of what control she can have over childbirth: Planning an epidural represents an attempt to ensure receipt of an anticipated beneficial intervention. As much faith as any mother might place in an epidural to improve her childbirth experience, the data herein show that she is still, to a greater or lesser extent, at the mercy of multiple forces outside her direct control. In particular, she is at the mercy of institutional readiness to administer the intervention she anticipates receiving. Furthermore, her labor progress must respond acceptably to intervention in order to remain within the professionally defined standard of 12 hours. She must also have an individual response to pain medication that matches standard dosage guidelines. Mothers in this chapter who met all the above criteria reported unequivocal satisfaction with childbirth, with the exception of Michelle, who gave a negative report on postpartum care.

In contrast, nearly all cases in which childbirth's physiological processes were either out of sync with institutional readiness or went astray of expectations of normalcy corresponded to qualified statements of maternal satisfaction. For five mothers with rapid labor progress, the primary force outside their control was a professional staff decision to proceed with unmedicated labor, violating the expectation of receiving an epidural and eliminating the related sense of control that went along with having planned the procedure in advance. Mothers whose labors exceeded the 12-hour mark not only had to contend with extra hours of hospital labor but were also exposed to a related series of caregiving events beyond their control—for example, Alana's requests for additional pain medication were met with apparent and frustrating inconsistency, and Marissa's nurse emphasized the possible negative consequences of vaginal (though apparently not cesarean) delivery.

Nonetheless, it must be restated that no mother, including those who had relatively short, unmedicated, and seemingly uncomplicated births and the one who reported an "epidural nightmare," expressed any postpartum negativity toward medical pain relief per se. Instead, these mothers appeared to wish they had benefited from quicker or more skilled administration or more effective pain relief, speaking perhaps to the allegiance one holds to a preconceived notion of the birth experience. Their ongoing interests also reflect many mothers' interest in—or, at the risk of stating it too strongly, fantasy of—powerful, maximally safe medical treatment for childbirth pain. Despite more than a century of dogged searching, an easily administered, fast-acting, long-lasting, side effect–free labor analgesia procedure effective for all women has yet to arrive, and very well may never come to be. Until such a solution is found, women deserve to know that epidural pain treatment is far from a perfect solution, and that institutional forces, each woman's own physiology, and the overall quality of obstetric care play important and related roles in how women ultimately view their childbirth experiences.

Chapter 5

Expectations and Experiences of Deferred Epidural Decisions

The Context of Deferring Epidural Decisions

Obstetric analgesia has become so deeply entrenched in the contemporary high-tech, low-touch U.S. birth culture as to engender a perception of on-demand availability. The epidural's perceived on-demand status allows mothers to consider laboring medication-free while having analgesia as a fall-back option should circumstances warrant it. Expecting to defer one's decision until some point in labor implies acceptance of the epidural as a definite option, distinguishing these mothers from naturally birthing women who opposed obstetric analgesia and from mothers who committed to analgesia well in advance of labor onset.

In my attempts to ascertain how frequently women plan for an epidural or defer their decisions on the procedure, I found no study addressing that specific question. In particular, no research appears to have been conducted on mothers who planned an epidural versus those who did not because they opposed the procedure (as in natural childbirth) and those who did not simply because they preferred to let circumstances guide their decisions. Thus, only inferences on the frequency and experiences of mothers expecting to "wait and see" on epidural could be drawn from related studies. For example, in one study, about 30% of pregnant women said they "didn't know" whether they wanted epidural, and another 3.5% said they "didn't care" (Impey, 1999); both responses presumably related to deferring decision making but are not exactly the same. Heinze and Sleigh (2003) found that only 10% of mothers who received epidural had not planned to have it in advance, but the authors did not distinguish whether mothers who had not planned epidural opposed it or delayed their decisions because they preferred to "wait and see."

Studies on the expectations and experiences of mothers expecting to "wait and see" whether to have an epidural were not available, but related work showed differences in maternal experiences as a function of planning or not planning the procedure. In one study distinguishing mothers' anticipation of epidural, 91% of women who stated during pregnancy that they "definitely" or "probably" would have an epidural went on to have one, whereas just over 50% of mothers who said they "hoped to avoid" or "did not intend" to have an epidural had one (Goldberg, Cohen, & Lieberman, 1999). A few other studies focused on satisfaction with childbirth, comparing groups of mothers who had planned epidural and those who had not. As one example, mothers who reported not wanting epidural prior to delivery but who later requested one reported lower pain than mothers who neither wanted nor had epidural, but those who had received epidural reported lower satisfaction, and most attributed dissatisfaction to having had an epidural (Kannan, Jamison, & Datta, 2001).

Whether maternal acceptance of or opposition to epidurals influences maternal satisfaction may be overshadowed by another important factor, which is the control mothers perceive in the decision to accept (or refuse) specific requested or recommended obstetric procedures. For example, a review of obstetric epidural studies revealed that pain relief as such did not strongly predict satisfaction with labor and delivery, but that "control variables," described as the mother's participation in decision making, did (Leeman, Fontaine, King, Klein, & Ratcliffe, 2003a, 2003b). Other researchers have worked toward refining the concept of maternal control, finding that a mother's perception of her control over staff actions toward her and her involvement in emergency and nonemergency obstetric decision making are important components in satisfaction with childbirth irrespective of interventions received (Green & Baston, 2003). Along similar lines, control—encompassing a sense of being at the center of and participating in the birth process and of maintaining personal authority and decision-making ability—related to childbirth satisfaction and a "good" birth experience; lack of control related to general dissatisfaction (Namey & Lyerly, 2010).

Because maternal control in obstetric decision making appears to be central to a mother's satisfaction with childbirth, it is worth examining the circumstances under which mothers might shift from a "wait and see" stance to accepting an epidural. The context in which mothers request or accept an epidural becomes especially important in light of the reality that in the hospital birth environment, obstetric professionals have greater power than laboring mothers. The power differential renders mothers vulnerable to pressure (or lack thereof) from obstetric professionals and places them at risk for dissatisfaction if conceding to professional pressure conflicts with their goals or desires (Wittmann-Price & Bhattacharya, 2008). Though many contemporary obstetric professionals and institutions promote "mother-centered" care in theory, obstetric analgesia produces income for hospitals, a reality that professionals have suggested at least partly underlies continually rising rates of epidural administration and associated obstetric interventions (Sakala, 2006).

The few available studies on the circumstances under which mothers shift from a "wait and see" stance on epidural to accepting the procedure have focused almost entirely on individual maternal factors rather than professional or situational variables. For example, in one of the few studies identifying a subgroup of mothers as "wait and see," women's reasons for changing from an initial perspective of "no epidural" or "wait and see" included labor induction, intense pain, protracted labor and exhaustion, anxiety about not knowing what to expect, perceived lack of control during labor, and inability to relax (Carlton, Callister, & Stoneman, 2005). Requests for epidural doubled among mothers who initially desired analgesia-free birth but whose labor duration exceeded 10 hours (Kannan et al., 2001). Rates of epidural requests among first-time mothers, for whom labor is a completely new experience, have been found to be up to five times higher than rates among multiparous mothers (K. Y. Chang, Chan, S. H. Chang, Yang, & Chen, 2008; Green & Baston, 2007).

In sum, a yet to be precisely determined percentage of mothers defers firmly deciding on or committing to epidural uptake but remains open to the procedure, a phenomenon I refer to as *deferring the decision*. A general lack of research in this area allows only inferences to be drawn on the expectations and experiences of mothers who expect to "wait and see." Maternal satisfaction may not necessarily be determined only by whether mothers expect to defer their analgesia decisions; also central may be whether they feel a sense of control over obstetric interventions that ultimately become part of their experiences. The circumstances under which a mother might shift from a "wait and see" stance may be important in related outcomes; extant research focuses primarily on maternal factors (e.g., labor pain, exhaustion) rather than on contextual factors as drivers of maternal decision making.

STUDY MOTHERS DEFERRING THE EPIDURAL DECISION

Ten (17%) vaginally birthing mothers were placed in this category based on their responses to a question on epidural indicating the expectation to defer deciding for or against the procedure until they had labored for a time. All except two mothers in this group were college educated, holding either an associate's or a bachelor's degree. Maternal ages ranged from 20 to 34 years. Two women reported family income in the poverty range, and the rest had middle-class incomes. Two mothers were non-white. All were married or had stable partners. Only one (10%) mother in this group was giving birth for the first time, whereas the remaining mothers were having their second or third children, and their previous deliveries had been vaginal. Following the approach outlined in chapter 1, I discuss findings for the whole group, illustrating them with quotes and examples of experiences drawn from select representative cases; mothers' names are fictional.

Expectations of Mothers Deferring the Epidural Decision

All 10 mothers in this group expected to have hospital vaginal delivery without an epidural, though all said they viewed the procedure as an option to be considered depending on circumstances. For example, 21-year-old first-time mother Desirae said that, like her own mother, she expected to labor medication-free but had discussed an epidural with her physician, who said she could change her mind up until four centimeters' dilation, so Desirae decided to keep the procedure "open as an option because I've never done this before, and I don't know what it will be like." Second-time mother Crystal, in her late 20s, said she had "talked about getting an epidural" with her obstetrician but emphasized that she was "not one who has to plan out … I'm kind of like, well, when the time comes … we'll go from there." Second-time mother Suzanne, who had an epidural with her first birth following labor induction, also intended to labor medication-free this time around but was "much more open" to the procedure than she had been previously.

Of all mothers in this group, second-time mother Renee stood out as the only one to defer her epidural decision because of concerns over rapid labor progress, which had precluded the procedure during her first birth. She said, "I don't know what I'm going to do when it comes down to pain medication. I didn't have an option … [with my first birth], so that's something I've really been thinking about and trying not to set too many standards."

Accompanying the expectation among this group's mothers to labor without an epidural was the anticipation of avoiding cesarean delivery;

the women held generally negative views toward the procedure. For example, first-time mother Desirae said, "I've seen it [cesarean delivery] done, and it's horrific ... I want to have another child ... if you have a c-section, it's hard to have another vaginal delivery." Like Desirae, Renee focused on surgical aspects of cesarean delivery in voicing her opposition to the procedure, saying, "I definitely want a vaginal birth."

In contrast to the uniform expectation of vaginal birth and avoidance of cesarean delivery, mothers' expectations of receiving other obstetric procedures varied. For example, none of the 10 mothers reported expecting to have labor induced, but one who had previously been induced said she "suspected" induction could become part of her upcoming experience. Half the mothers did, however, say they would prefer having labor induced to waiting for natural labor onset if their pregnancies were to pass the due date by a week or so; those favoring induction focused primarily on concern about large fetal size. Echoing a sentiment shared by four other mothers, Maria said, "I don't want it to get any bigger than it has to be."

Mothers in this group uniformly expected electronic fetal monitoring. However, five of the nine experienced mothers neither expected nor found acceptable internal monitoring. Crystal expressed the strongest objection, saying, "My husband and I ... would not allow that."

No mother mentioned expectation of analgesia-related complications for herself or her newborn. Mothers did not, unless prompted, mention any expectation of other widely used obstetric procedures, such as labor acceleration or episiotomy. With prompting, mothers generally expressed uncertainty about whether to expect labor acceleration (drugs or amniotomy), though none expressed any particular opposition. No mother expected systemic analgesia, but two mothers said they felt "fine" about it if it became necessary, shown in Amy's statement, "What the mom wants, that's OK." Two other mothers expressed clear opposition to intravenous (IV) analgesia, and the remaining mothers were unsure. Mothers did not expect instrumental delivery, and were generally opposed to it, though one did say she found instrumental assistance acceptable "if necessary." No mother said she expected episiotomy.

Expectations Mentioned Less Frequently

Among their childbirth expectations, four mothers mentioned an uncomplicated birth. All these mothers had previously given birth with what they referred to as no or minor complications—with the exception of Suzanne, who had been in good health throughout her current pregnancy but had been diagnosed with preeclampsia with her firstborn. In contrast, three mothers mentioned expecting complications either based on information they had received during the current pregnancy or because they had previously experienced a complicated birth. For example, first-time mother Desirae's physician had told her she had "borderline diabetes" and had mentioned that she could be a "candidate for a c-section." Amy, too, worried most about possible cesarean delivery because "right now, the baby is not head down. If my water breaks and the baby would be in a funky position, then I would have to have a cesarean."

With experience as their guide, subgroups of mothers who had previously given birth raised additional expectations relative to their previous labors. Two mothers said they expected a birth experience better than a previous one. Maria preferred to have her "kids natural," which to her meant medication-free, but having previously endured two long medication-free labors, she was keeping her mind open to "whatever my doctor does to keep me comfortable." Crystal had received an epidural in her previous birth but expected to have more say about the timing and the dosage if she accepted the procedure this time around; she preferred to experience relief but not total pain block as she had previously, which she found "frustrating" because she did not "know when to push."

Three experienced mothers explicitly referred to expecting a specific labor duration, which for all happened to be short. Renee, for example, reflected on her general labor and delivery expectations, saying, "I think it's going to go really fast … that's all I can say. My son was born in three and a half hours." Similarly, Amy said her only firm childbirth expectation was to "dilate very quickly."

Consistent with statements by mothers in other vaginally birthing groups, two of this group's experienced mothers referred to not knowing what to anticipate. For example, Maria said she "had no idea" what to expect. Suzanne, whose previous labor had been induced, said she felt excited about "going into labor naturally" but that given the surprises that accompanied her previous birth, she had "learned not to" hold firm expectations, adding, "Knowing what to expect doesn't make it any easier for me."

Three mothers in this group mentioned expecting pain or discomfort in their upcoming births; first-time mother Desirae mentioned pain first among her expectations, and Maria said she expected "to be uncomfortable."

GREATEST FEARS IN CHILDBIRTH

To elicit other expectations mothers might have not revealed upon direct questioning, I asked, "What is your greatest worry about your upcoming birth?" Two of the three mothers who said they expected pain also mentioned pain as their greatest worry; Suzanne's concern about "the pain of it ripping out of me" was the most explicit. Two other mothers mentioned cesarean delivery as their greatest worry, stated most strongly by Crystal: "I hope I never have to have one."

Other mothers based their childbirth concerns on previous experience. Suzanne, diagnosed with preeclampsia in a previous birth, worried about the condition "coming back." Maria, who said her previous labors had been long, was most concerned that labor and delivery would "just take too long." Renee, the only mother in this group to defer her decision on an epidural because of concerns about rapidly progressing labor, said she worried most about getting to the hospital in time for delivery, partly to avoid frightening her toddler with a possible "emergency situation." With the exception of Suzanne's concern over a recurrence of preeclampsia, no other mother in this group mentioned concerns about her own health. One mother mentioned concern over newborn health, saying she worried most about having "a healthy baby."

Summary of Expectations in Mothers Deferring the Epidural Decision

The 10 mothers in this group, nine of whom had previously given birth, shared the expectation of attempting labor and delivery without medication but also the anticipation that epidural would be available during labor if they felt the circumstances warranted it. All shared the expectation of vaginal birth, consistent with the related expressed desire to avoid cesarean delivery. Reflecting the general view that epidural procedures are available on demand, only two mothers mentioned concerns over analgesia availability; one mother focused on medical practices that limit the procedure's availability and the other focused on the possibility that her own labor progress might preclude its administration. No mother expected induced labor or episiotomy, whereas all expected external fetal monitoring. No mother expected internal fetal monitoring, and several mothers strongly opposed it. Mothers generally expressed uncertain expectations about other widely used obstetric procedures, such as labor-accelerating drugs and amniotomy. Some, though not all, mothers referred to expecting an uncomplicated birth, a better birth experience than previous ones, a short labor duration, and (consistent with other vaginally birthing mothers) childbirth pain. Mothers' greatest childbirth fears related primarily to specific aspects of the birth experience, including extremely short or long labor duration or possible cesarean delivery.

Confirmed and Violated Expectations in Mothers Deferring the Decision

This group's shared expectations of going into labor naturally, of laboring for a time without analgesia, and of delivering vaginally were confirmed for four (40%). Four (40%) mothers' expectations of natural labor onset were violated by labor induction. Three mothers' expectations of vaginal delivery were violated with cesarean delivery. One mother had an episiotomy. Of mothers who experienced expectancy violations, two encountered single violations and the other four, multiple violations.

Of the four mothers who experienced multiple expectancy violations, two developed gestational diabetes (Desirae, Maria) in late pregnancy. Suzanne was not formally diagnosed with preeclampsia but had an abnormal blood-pressure reading and was treated in a manner consistent with a preeclampsia diagnosis. The two mothers with gestational diabetes both delivered by cesarean. All 10 mothers received some form of labor analgesia: Eight received an epidural, one received general anesthesia, and one mother received systemic analgesia only. All mothers reported effective pain relief; descriptions ranged from "taking the edge off" to "no pain at all; it was wonderful."

Cases of Confirmed Expectations

Renee, who had avoided firmly committing to an epidural because of concerns about rapid labor progress, said childbirth this time was "right on, actually." Once labor started, Renee went to the hospital but she said staff turned her away and she "had to walk around" for about an hour, a practice consistent with true active-labor-management protocols that recommend hospitals admit mothers only after active labor has begun, theoretically reducing maternal stress and the related potential for "stalled" labor in the hospital (Boylan, 1989). About two hours after being admitted, Renee accepted an offer of epidural, had the procedure, and "three contractions later," her newborn arrived. Renee said she was glad she had an epidural because it allowed her to "participate a little more" in those three contractions. By Renee's description, the offer of an epidural came before she had firmly decided to have one because her labor was progressing so quickly. After the fact, one can only wonder whether Renee would have requested the procedure had it not been offered, especially if she had been offered lower risk, nonmedical pain relief, such as water or massage. Moreover, though epidurals are associated with slower labor, the procedure hardly seemed to slow Renee's labor. In fact, her rapid labor progress upon hospital admission resulted in an unexpected surprise stemming from hospital protocol. With a diagnosed group B streptococcus (GBS) infection, she was to undergo intrapartum antibiotic prophylaxis (IAP) during labor. Unfortunately, her full antibiotic course could not be administered during her short labor, so she and her newborn had to remain hospitalized an extra day to, in Renee's words, "keep an eye on the baby," which she found upsetting because of additional costs.

Like Renee's, Crystal's generally confirmed childbirth expectations met with an unanticipated event related to hospital protocol. Crystal said she "independently decided on" an epidural well before reporting to the hospital in active labor, and she labored there for about six hours. She had an epidural and felt ready to push about 90 minutes later. However, Crystal said hospital staff discouraged her from doing so because the attending physician was not due to arrive for another 30 minutes. "They were going to give me more drugs," Crystal said, but she refused. Staff continued to pressure her, so she enlisted her husband's help in asserting her wishes:

> It was kind of difficult when I was dilated to a ten; we didn't want to have to wait for the actual doctor to come … it took quite a bit of convincing to tell them we didn't want to wait, we're just going to have the resident deliver.

As unsettling as I found Renee's being offered an epidural as an apparent first-line treatment when she was a mere three contractions away from delivery, I found Crystal's account of being told to resist the instinctual urge to push and accept more medication for institutional convenience deeply disturbing. Fortunately, though she was under the stress of labor, Crystal took the necessary steps to move forward and delivered without complications. Her newborn did, however, arrive "very jaundiced." Several weeks after discharge, the baby was rehospitalized for respiratory distress syndrome and contracted pneumonia in the hospital, where she stayed almost two weeks; but Crystal reported that "they think she'll grow out of it … she's doing a lot better now."

Case of Single Expectancy Violation

Amy's expectation of natural labor onset was violated with labor induction, but she described labor and delivery itself as "exactly how I thought it would be." Amy said she believed her water had broken "in the car, of all places," so she reported to the hospital. Contractions had not begun, and staff attempted to initiate the process by administering oxytocin, which triggered mild contractions, but she "wasn't dilating." To move things along, Amy said, medical staff broke what she called a "floor bag" that was blocking the cervix and preventing full-on labor. Having earlier decided against an epidural, at this point Amy accepted "some drugs," specifically, IV opiates. An internal fetal monitor was placed for reasons Amy said she did not understand. "Four, maybe eight" hours later, Amy said, her newborn arrived with a "big ol' scratch" on the scalp from the internal/intravaginal monitor, leading Amy to remark on not understanding "why they had to do that." It is plausible that internal monitoring was used as a matter of protocol given reported concerns about IV opiates' potential effects on fetal heart rate and responsiveness (Reynolds, 2010).

Cases of Multiple Expectancy Violations

Desirae, who had been diagnosed with gestational diabetes late in pregnancy, said she suspected cesarean delivery "would probably happen" owing to concerns about large fetal size. Even so, she proceeded with a plan for vaginal birth and had labor induced as scheduled, about a week before her newborn's due date. Labor was induced in the evening, and after sleeping on and off and asking to "prolong the labor" throughout the following day to maximize her chances of delivering vaginally, Desirae received late afternoon news of her fetus's "heart rate lowering," at which point cesarean delivery was "strongly suggested." Desirae felt she "didn't really have a choice" because she worried about fetal safety. Surgery ensued, and Desirae's baby arrived safely by 6:30 p.m. Though she cast her overall experience as "kind of" what she expected, Desirae found herself surprised by nurses whom she described as "mean" and by effects of the surgery:

> I couldn't walk, couldn't stand … I couldn't deal [with] … showers [or with] … lying down … [It was] horrible. I was on pain medications, but it really didn't really work … A couple months

> later I tried to do some stretches and it opened, the surface, and I started to bleed … it still hurts.

At 6 pounds, 2 ounces, Desirae's baby weighed considerably less than supposed in the rationale for scheduling her induction a week early, and that initial procedure led to the same cascade of interventions ending in cesarean that has been recounted by other mothers in this book.

Like Desirae, Maria had gestational diabetes and had been forewarned about large fetal size (her newborn weighed 5 pounds, 1 ounce). However, she did not have any expectation or suspicion that she might deliver by cesarean. About a month before her due date, Maria's water broke, and she went to the hospital. Admissions staff judiciously sent Marie home because she "wasn't dilating at all" and advised her to return the next morning. When she returned, Maria said she had high blood pressure and her fetus's heart rate was "really high."

> They … put me to sleep … It wasn't anything I ever expected … I don't really remember him being born … The doctor told me that … I had really no choice. The baby was stressed and I was [too] … he just went with what was best for both … something that had to be done. I was freaking out, just crying; I was pretty scared. I didn't get to do anything.

Just as she did not understand exactly what had led to the emergency cesarean, Maria also did not fully understand why her newborn was immediately hospitalized in the NICU postpartum, though she believed he had contracted an infection. Maria's native language is not English, and I became concerned about what role that may have played in her communication with staff. Maria did not say much when I asked how she felt about her communication with staff, but she did report that her newborn was now healthy and doing well.

In Suzanne's case, previous experience with complications arising from a pregnancy condition did little to prepare her for a complicated childbirth trajectory that arose more from institutional issues than from her physical condition or the birth process. Suzanne said that her blood pressure was creeping upward with each prenatal visit, and though she was not formally diagnosed with preeclampsia, her physician treated her as if she had been and scheduled labor induction two weeks before Suzanne's due date. About "five minutes" before she was to leave her home for the hospital, Suzanne said, staff called and told her the hospital was full, encouraging her to report to an alternate hospital rather than wait for an available slot. Suzanne then contacted her doctor who advised her to go to the alternate hospital because she was going to "be out of town" a few days later. Suzanne reported to the alternate hospital, which she described as smaller, less comfortable, and generally aversive, saying, "You can't argue anything … I hated them there. I hated it." Her induction was slow to "take," and the next morning, her physician broke her water, which Suzanne believed was "an accident," adding that she had not wanted that. (In the context of having her induction rescheduled apparently to meet physician convenience, I wondered how much of an accident the amniotomy had been.) Labor proceeded quickly, but her epidural was delayed because the anesthesiologist arrived several hours after Suzanne had made the request. Her baby arrived safely a few hours later, but Suzanne still felt "really upset … [because] the whole hospital and the way they do everything was way different than what I wanted."

SATISFACTION

Maternal reports on satisfaction with the overall childbirth experience were decidedly mixed in this group; mothers who had either no or a single expectancy violation reported that they were "satisfied," "pretty satisfied," or "very satisfied." Second-time mother Amy, who did not receive epidural but did have systemic analgesia, gave the least qualified response to the satisfaction question, saying, "Everything went pretty much the way I wanted it to … It was a very positive experience" with the exception of the unwanted internal monitoring. Amy attributed her positive responses to the facts that the same nurse stayed with her for the duration of her labor and that she had not received an epidural; she said this allowed her greater ability to control her urges to push. In fact, Amy said, she "highly" recommended "not getting epidurals."

Other mothers whose expectations were confirmed nonetheless qualified their satisfaction statements. For example, Renee, whose labor and delivery proceeded practically problem free, said she was "very satisfied" with the overall experience. Because she had received IAP in advanced labor and had to pay for a longer than anticipated hospital stay, she also wished she had been "more forceful" about getting herself admitted to the hospital; she felt that nursing staff "wouldn't listen to me that I was in labor." Generally, the true active-labor-management guideline for admitting mothers to hospital only after active labor has begun works to everyone's benefit, but in Renee's case, what many would have considered an enviably brief obstetric hospitalization turned into a longer one because of the hospital's IAP administration routine. The other mother whose birth experience generally confirmed expectations, Crystal, also faced institutional protocol when she felt ready to deliver before the attending physician had arrived. Crystal expressed some ambivalence over having had an epidural, as well: "I wish I wouldn't have, but it definitely felt better once it was in there ... it went a lot smoother than the first time when I attempted to get an epidural." Even so, Crystal said she felt "pretty satisfied" overall. It is worth noting that both these mothers shared another feature in their birth experience: They labored in the hospital considerably less than 12 hours each.

Mothers who experienced multiple expectancy violations also had pregnancy issues that one might surmise would complicate their birth experiences and their related satisfaction. In Desirae's case, earlier awareness or suspicion that cesarean delivery could occur may have buffered against greater negativity, shown in her report of feeling, overall, "pretty satisfied." But Desirae also said that things "could have gone better" and went on to describe wishing staff had spent more time explaining her pain medications and their effects as they were progressively administered. Maria, who had previously delivered two children vaginally and had no previous awareness or suspicion that cesarean birth could become part of her experience, simply "didn't know" whether she was satisfied. Her later statements did suggest lingering negativity, however, for she went on to say she wished she had "looked into" cesarean delivery beforehand, adding, "You don't ever think it could happen to you, but it's something that's just all of a sudden … I wish I had … really looked into that before."

Suzanne separated the experience of giving birth itself from her treatment, describing the former as "great," and the latter as leaving her "unsatisfied," a sentiment stemming from the last-minute change in her hospital. Suzanne's tale of institutionally driven changes to her birth expectations and her discussion of staff behavior reinforced why she would have been unsatisfied or worse. She closed her story by saying, "When I was in labor, she [an obstetric nurse] was talking about my high blood pressure … I'm overweight … She said … if I wanted to live … I'd better do something about my blood pressure. She was just harassing me … I [hadn't] even had the baby yet."

Summary and Implications

Mothers in this group distinguished themselves by expressing an expectation of laboring for an indeterminate length of time before firmly deciding whether to request an epidural. These mothers also expected natural labor onset, vaginal delivery, fetal monitoring, and no instruments or episiotomy. Once in labor, nine mothers decided to accept labor analgesia (eight epidural, one systemic), and the tenth had general anesthesia administered before emergency cesarean delivery. The uptake and availability of epidural for the eight mothers who accepted it confirmed the procedure's status as available "on demand." Even with apparently readily available epidural and across-the-board effectiveness reported among this group's mothers, childbirth expectations were fully confirmed for only four (40%) women. Two mothers had single expectancy violations, and the remaining four had multiple expectancy violations that, in three cases, started with labor induction and ended with cesarean delivery.

The majority of women in the previous chapter's formal planning group and in this chapter's deferring group subsequently underwent the epidural procedure, making the primary distinction between the two subsets the language mothers used to describe their expectations. Mothers planning epidural explicitly stated an expectation of a procedure in our interviews while they were pregnant, and in nearly all cases they had reportedly made or intended to make their expectations known to some obstetric professional. In contrast, mothers in the deferring group made explicit only their expectations of keeping epidural open as an option and, by their reports, had not made any expressed commitment to obstetric professionals.

Whether the language mothers used to describe their expectations reflected any real difference in underlying intentions remains an open question with no likely definitive answers. General ambivalence toward epidural (and other) labor analgesia characterizes contemporary birth culture; proponents point to a maternal right to obstetric pain relief and overall analgesia safety, and opponents point to analgesia's variable effects and possible, sometimes serious, consequences. Historical records of maternal and fetal death and disability from unsafe obstetric pain treatment, of deeply rooted (though not necessarily consciously felt) religious proscriptions against treating childbirth pain, and of cultural value placed on individual strength further complicate some women's views on any form of obstetric pain relief. In such a context, some mothers may find it more personally and socially acceptable to adopt a "wait and see" stance rather than plainly stating, in advance, commitment to procedures shrouded in controversy.

Although epidural uptake rates among both mothers who planned epidural and mothers who deferred the decision were nearly identical, childbirth expectations were confirmed for almost 20% fewer mothers in the deferring group. This result could easily be an artifact of the relatively small numbers of women in either group. It could also relate to the relatively high percentage (30%) of mothers in the deferring group who developed risk or borderline risk in late pregnancy and whose births subsequently became more complicated, necessitating more medical intervention and the related loss of control their reports suggest.

Mothers' reports in this chapter and in previous chapters evidence a dynamic process involving multiple factors in ultimate childbirth expectancy confirmation or violation. Certainly, maternal physical factors played a role, and a hospital labor duration of less than 12 hours generally triggered the fewest unanticipated responses in relation to institutional protocols and the individuals administering them. Shorter hospital labor duration does not, however, translate into freedom from unanticipated institutional intrusion. For example, of those mothers featured in this chapter, Renee and Crystal reported straightforward and rapid labor progress, analgesia administered at their request, and effective pain relief, but both mothers encountered unexpected (and unwelcome) surprises related to mandated hospital stay and staff requirements for newborn delivery, respectively. Subsequently, both mothers reported general satisfaction with their otherwise largely confirmed childbirth expectations, but they qualified their statements with reference to those unanticipated intrusions.

In contrast, Desirae, Maria, and Suzanne started down a path towards violated childbirth expectations once identified risk or near risk arose in their pregnancies. Given their risk status, some childbirth expectancy violation involving a particular obstetric procedure might have been predicted for all three mothers, as in, for example, Maria's report of emergency cesarean delivery. However, considerably more difficult to predict would have been the manner in which those interventions were delivered, the level of reported maternal control in the process, and accompanying staff behavior. For example, one might have predicted that Suzanne would have experienced induced labor, but few would (or could) have foreseen the last-minute hospital change she reported, its apparent relationship to her physician's availability, and Suzanne's related negative views on the overall experience. These examples show that physical risk alone is only part of the childbirth expectancy confirmation or violation process and only one of several forces limiting or eradicating any maternal role in obstetric decision making.

Overall, virtually no difference between the availability or uptake of obstetric analgesia was evidenced between groups of mothers planning or deferring epidural decisions. More mothers in the deferring group, however, had their childbirth expectations violated, and violations occurred through a process involving factors mostly outside direct maternal control—primarily, their physical status, related institutional responses, and what came across as their diminished role in decision making. Although mothers whose hospital labor time unfolds in less than 12 hours appear to risk fewer unanticipated (and usually unwelcome) institutional intrusions or negative staff responses, "normal" labor duration by no means guarantees an unqualified, satisfactory childbirth experience from the maternal perspective. Based on this chapter's maternal reports, routine institutional practices designed to enhance maternal and fetal safety, such as labor induction and cesarean surgery, violate maternal expectations in their practice, their consequences, and the manner in which they are administered.

Chapter 6

Expectations and Experiences of Planned Cesarean Delivery

The Context of Planned Cesarean Delivery

Cesarean or *c-section delivery* likely takes its name not from Julius Caesar but from one of his earlier ancestors who reportedly survived being cut from his mother's abdomen after her death in childbirth (Lurie, 2005). Though cross-cultural accounts of surgically delivering neonates from deceased mothers date back more than 2,500 years, and European physicians attempted cesarean delivery on live women as early as the 16th century (Graham, 1951), only in the past few decades has planning surgical delivery to occur in advance of labor become more widespread. Because of its relatively recent arrival on the childbirth scene and variable definitions of what constitutes "planned" cesarean delivery, statistics on the procedure vary. As a rough estimate, U.S. statistics show that about half of early 21st-century's U.S. total cesarean births were planned, most of them on women who had previously had one or more cesareans

(Declercq, Menacker, & MacDorman, 2006; MacDorman, Menacker, & Declercq, 2008; Menacker, Declercq, & MacDorman, 2006; Menacker & Hamilton, 2010). The other half of the total cesareans, about 32% of all births in the early 21st-century United States, were the perhaps more familiar labored or emergency cesarean.

In general, planned cesarean birth involves scheduling abdominal delivery on or near a mother's due date so that she can avoid going into labor, reflecting a preference to accept surgical risks over those of labor in certain situations. For example, laboring with a fetus in the breech position (the fetus enters the birth canal feet or rump first rather than head first) is riskier for both mother and child than the normal vertex (head down) position. Labor with multiple fetuses can become complicated, particularly if one or more fetuses is positioned unfavorably for birth (Cunningham et al., 2009). But by far the most common reason for planning cesarean delivery is to prevent labor-related risks resulting from one or more previous cesareans: Very rarely, uterine scars from previous cesarean births can rupture during labor. In the United States, planned cesarean delivery has become the treatment of choice in these and other pregnancy situations based less on convincing scientific research and more on a "dogmatic belief that cesarean section may … improve perinatal outcome" (Schachar & Weinstein, 1998, p. 447). Few large-scale clinical studies of cesarean delivery in certain higher risk situations have been conducted, particularly in the United States, where such practice is becoming routine in the absence of convincing clinical evidence. In contrast, studies conducted in Canada and Europe have shown that vaginal delivery in breech and twin birth can be advantageous for both mothers and neonates (e.g., Daskalakis et al., 2007; Su et al., 2007); similar findings on the advantages of planned vaginal delivery after cesarean are reviewed in chapter 7.

Once decided on, planned cesarean delivery proceeds much like the emergency cesarean surgical procedure from which it was derived and carries similar risks. After administering epidural analgesia or anesthesia, the surgeon begins a 45- to 90-minute procedure involving cutting through the abdomen just above the pubic bone, pulling apart muscles, and cutting through the uterus. Amniotic fluid is suctioned out; the surgeon pulls the baby head first through the openings, removes the placenta and membranes, stitches up the uterus, repositions internal parts, and closes the cut (Cunningham et al., 2009). Women do not generally report pain, but they may report pressure, tugging, and stitching sensations. After centuries of learning about human physiology and surgical techniques, cesarean delivery has become highly advanced, assuming the position of the most common in-hospital surgery among U.S. women (Hall, DeFrances, Williams, Golosinskiy, & Schwartzman, 2010).

Planned or labored cesarean reduces certain labor risks, but it also comes with drawbacks. Like any surgery, cesarean delivery poses the usual risks of analgesia or anesthesia and surgical cutting; however, full understanding of those risks in planned cesareans has yet to be achieved. Much of the research comparing vaginal and cesarean delivery has been conducted on labored cesarean over the past 30 years. Not only have anesthesia and surgical techniques advanced in those years, but because planned cesarean is performed on a body that has not undergone the stress of labor, its outcomes will presumably differ from those of labored cesarean. Long-term effects on maternal or newborn health of skipping labor altogether remain largely unknown. Moreover, planned cesarean is theoretically performed to address a maternal or fetal health concern, so comparing these deliveries to vaginal births is akin to comparing the proverbial apples and oranges.

Even so, certain risks of planned cesarean surgery are fairly clear. Because the uterus itself is cut, subsequent scarring creates risks for future pregnancies and births (Jackson & Paterson-Brown, 2001). Other consequences may occur in vaginal birth as well but arise less frequently because vaginal birth does not involve anesthesia and surgery. For example, thromboembolism (serious blood clot) occurs 2 to 20 times more frequently in planned or labored cesarean than in vaginal birth because surgery can cause blood loss, dehydration, and problems stemming from immobility (NIH, 2006). Placental abnormalities, potentially harmful to mothers and fetuses, occur in about 5% of women who have never delivered by cesarean compared to 24% of women with one previous cesarean and 47% of those with two (Jackson & Paterson-Brown, 2001). Cesarean surgery can cost up to twice as much financially as vaginal birth (Declercq et al., 2007). Maternal death may occur up to three times more frequently in labored cesarean than in vaginal birth (Hall & Bewley, 1999), but planned cesarean maternal mortality data remain inconclusive (NIH, 2006).

Other complications of cesarean delivery do not develop with vaginal birth. Abdominal surgical suture ruptures and surgical wound infections occur during hospitalization in an estimated 3–9% of cesarean cases (Jackson & Paterson-Brown, 2001). Up to 20% of mothers see physicians in outpatient visits for surgical wound infections. In vaginal birth, passing through the birth canal helps kick-start the neonatal respiratory system; cesarean surgery bypasses that process, thus putting the newborn at risk for breathing and associated respiratory problems and postpartum special care or NICU hospitalization (Cunningham et al., 2009; Donahue et al., 1994). Early breathing problems may continue, translating into higher rates of childhood asthma. Unintended neonatal lacerations resulting from the surgery, usually minor, may also occur (Geller, Wu, Jannelli, Nguyen, & Visco, 2010).

Studies on cesarean's psychological effects tend to involve small numbers of women; broad statements about delivery mode as a source of maternal distress are further complicated by when, how, and to whom women report their symptoms. Several studies have found that women with labored cesareans report higher rates of postpartum childbirth trauma symptoms (Olde, van der Hart, Kleber, & van Son, 2006). Maternal history of psychiatric instability, perceptions of poor staff treatment, perceived lack of control, and ongoing pain, however, appear to trigger postpartum trauma and depressive symptoms as powerfully as cesarean surgery itself (Carter et al., 2006; Eisenach et al., 2008). Successful breastfeeding most often begins immediately postpartum, but the process can be complicated by cesarean-related maternal surgical recovery and related fatigue and abdominal discomfort; cesarean delivery has therefore been clearly associated with lower breastfeeding rates and shorter breastfeeding duration (NIH, 2006). Maternal surgical recovery may also compromise the quality of early mother-infant attachment, and compromised early attachment quality may negatively affect attachment quality in later infancy and beyond.

In sum, the nature and degree of risk associated with cesarean surgery depends on the medical indications for the surgery and on whether a cesarean is planned or labored; the latter is associated with greater risks. Fully understanding planned cesarean benefits and risks will require a system-wide, coordinated effort. In the absence of high-quality, long-term studies, which one would hope form the basis for medical decision making, determining appropriate circumstances for planned cesarean is something of a judgment call. Put simply, even when obstetric professionals want to abide by acceptable standards for practice, no definitive standards exist.

Until definitive data to guide cesarean decisions are reported—something that may or may not occur—mothers remain in the midst of complex forces that appear to be driving planned and labored cesarean surgery rates steadily upward from the current U.S. rate of 32%, amounting to more than 1.25 million births every year (MacDorman et al., 2008). Some have questioned whether an increasingly unhealthy and older maternal population for whom vaginal birth is actually riskier than cesarean surgery is responsible the upward trend (Ecker & Frigoletto, 2007). Planned cesarean births are higher in so-called high-risk mothers, but rates are also rising in all industrialized nations among healthy mothers (Betrán et al., 2007). Others have referred to women's overt requests for planned cesarean delivery, formally referred to as *cesarean delivery on maternal request* (CDMR), a controversial proposition that the U.S. National Institutes of Health examined with an expert panel in 2006. After reviewing reliable data sources, the panel concluded that fewer than 5% of women overtly requested cesarean delivery without any medical reason (e.g., Gamble & Creedy, 2000; Gamble, Creedy, McCourt, Weaver, & Beake, 2007); it is therefore best to say that CDMR occurs infrequently.

According to available statistics, the primary driver of increasing planned cesarean numbers is repeat cesarean surgery (Menacker & Hamilton, 2010), which was the case for 81% of the mothers featured in this chapter. Vaginal birth after cesarean (VBAC) became more common in the early 1990s, and the U.S. cesarean surgery rate actually fell (see chapter 7). VBAC steadily fell out of favor following a rekindling of concerns about uterine rupture. Uterine rupture can occur in vaginal birth, but labor contractions stress the uterus, and cesarean surgery–induced thinning and scarring create further risk. Thus, previous cesareans account for over 90% of uterine rupture incidents (Kieser & Baskett, 2002). Though uterine rupture occurs in fewer than 1 in 1,000 births and the most severe consequences—maternal or neonatal death—are even rarer, uterine rupture remains among obstetrics professionals' greatest fears.

One cannot dismiss how powerfully a cultural fear of childbirth's going terribly awry—no matter how remote the possibility—has influenced childbirth practices in the United States and elsewhere. As physicians perform more cesarean surgeries under the belief that the benefits outweigh the risks, they become more confident and increasingly view the procedure as routine and safe while at the same time becoming less comfortable with, for example, VBAC. Along with fear of childbirth complications comes fear of lawsuits, and practicing obstetricians reported "fear of litigation" as the primary reason for their performing more cesareans than they did five or ten years ago (Clark, Belfort, Byrum, Myers, & Perlin, 2008; Clark, Belfort, Dildy, & Myers, 2008). In addition, robust evidence indicates increased cesarean delivery rates alongside available institutional resources to support the surgery (Lauer, Betrán, Merialdi, & Wojdyla, 2010).[1]

STUDY MOTHERS ANTICIPATING PLANNED CESAREAN DELIVERY

Of the 75 mothers in this study, 16 (21%) were planning cesarean. Thirteen (81%) were repeat cesareans following a previous labored cesarean or, in one case, a previous planned cesarean. Two women were first-time mothers expecting twins. One was a first-time mother with a vaguely described medical indication. Mothers' education ranged from less than high school to master's degree, and income ranged from poverty level to upper middle-class income. Four mothers were nonwhite. Five mothers had public health insurance. Fourteen were married or had stable partners; the other two had inconsistent contact with or support from partners. Ten (62%) held part- or full-time employment outside the home. Following the approach outlined in chapter 1, I discuss findings for the whole group, citing quotes and examples of experiences drawn from select representative cases; mothers' names are fictional.

Mothers described a combination of factors—including their own preferences, physician input, and institutional requirements—as influencing their decisions to plan cesarean delivery, and the relative influence of each factor varied case by case. For example, both mothers of twins described an initial preference for vaginal birth, but they took physician input to heart and scheduled surgery at 37 weeks' pregnancy to prevent complications, a stance captured in Heather's statement, "[The doctor] let me know … you could push and push and push and still end up with a c-section … she wanted me to know all the possibilities … my best-case scenario … [both babies would] probably [be] breeched … which can cause all kinds of other problems." Heather made no mention of her physician's describing surgical risks, physical or otherwise. First-time mother Gemma said she feared vaginal delivery, mentioning concerns that her small size would make childbirth difficult. She reported discussing her interest in cesarean delivery with her doctor, saying, "My doctor actually wants to schedule me for a c-section 'cause he thinks my pelvis bone is gonna break … he's … really serious … I'm really little, and he's scared my hips won't open." Gemma, like Heather, made no mention of her physician's presenting the risks of cesarean delivery.

Like Heather and Gemma, 11 mothers indicated that their own preferences and professional medical input had combined to influence their decisions to plan cesarean delivery, though in these 11 cases the decision was to repeat cesarean surgery following a previous one. For example, Ana, whose previous 20-some-hour hospital labor had concluded with cesarean birth, said she "actually preferred" cesarean delivery and readily went along with her physician's recommendation to "have the c-section" based on his concerns that her placenta could have placed itself on her previous surgical scar. Fourth-time mother Debra said she, too, preferred cesarean delivery after having delivered her firstborn vaginally because "I don't do well with pain that way … there's nothing that really helps that actual labor process." Debra did, however, resent medical pressure to schedule cesarean, saying, "Sometimes nurses will come in and go, 'Do you want a c-section?' And it's like, well, you're just [now] asking me. Let me think about it for a while … Take one step at a time." Along similar lines, second-time mother Ivey said she "kind of preferred" cesarean delivery because she "knew what to expect." However, Ivey also gave the impression that cesarean delivery was expected of her, saying, "They just schedule it and go … In most places … [for] insurance reasons, if you had one c-section, they make you get another one. It's because of the state."

Among the two mothers who would have preferred VBAC, Sharon said her obstetric clinic offered her no choice because her previous cesarean had involved a vertical rather than horizontal surgical cut (vertical cuts are more likely to rupture), leading her to say, "Darn, something is wrong with me. That stinks. I wish I could do it … but it's not in the cards for me." Mei, who had initially planned VBAC because she wanted to continue with her clinic's midwife, said a "borderline" gestational diabetes test result had led to recommended planned cesarean. She went along with the recommendation, but Mei remained "on the fence" about the decision, largely because it conflicted with her immigrant mother's views: "They don't believe in doing any kind of surgery that's not essential … my mother was furious with me … she thought it was too dangerous."

Expectations of Planned Cesarean Delivery

Because planned cesarean delivery is a treatment package designed to bypass the labor process entirely, mothers' expressed expectations of childbirth are necessarily constrained to components of the surgical delivery plan. Expectations in terms of, for example, when or how labor might begin, how long it might last, types of pain medication, and whether cesarean birth will occur have all been predetermined. Under the assumption of avoiding labor with planned cesarean delivery, most (14; 88%) but not all study mothers shared the expectation of no labor. Of the two mothers who expected natural labor onset, Tasha, expecting twins, said she suspected labor would begin prematurely and before her scheduled surgical date. Ivey stated her expectation of natural labor onset in direct terms, "I do believe my water's going to break and they're going to have to do an emergency c-section, like they did with [my firstborn]; my water broke, and he went into distress."

No labor was the expectation shared among the most mothers in this group; the second-most frequently mentioned expectation was shared among 12 mothers: a short time to delivery. For example, Heather, expecting twins, anticipated arriving at the hospital and delivering her newborns "before noon." Mei, who had previously labored about five hours following an induction that ended in labored cesarean, expected her planned cesarean to "go fast," and she looked forward to a short wait before meeting her newborn. Debra, who had previously delivered twins by planned cesarean, expected an even "more relaxed" and shorter time to delivery than previously.

Most mothers undergoing repeat cesarean mentioned knowing what to expect, a sentiment captured in Sharon's words, "I think I pretty much know what to expect." Nine other mothers undergoing repeat cesarean referred specifically to their previous surgeries as the basis for knowing what to expect.

Less Frequently Mentioned Expectations

In contrast to the short wait time 12 mothers expected, two mothers expected long wait times for surgery. For example, Ivey said she expected "a lot of waiting in the hospital, a lot of boredom."

Two mothers referred specifically to pain-related expectations, but in contrasting ways. Gemma said she expected childbirth pain but remembered her physician's saying, "When you get a c-section, there'll be a lot of medicine that keep[s] you numb, and you don't feel anything." In contrast, Carolyn's previous experience with an epidural that effectively blocked labor pain and surgical sensations led her to expect to have "no feeling at all" in her planned repeat cesarean delivery.

Other expectations were mentioned only one time each. Heather, a first-time mother, said she generally did not have "a lot of expectations." Carolyn expected some difficulty dealing with family members anxious to meet the newborn.

GREATEST FEARS IN CHILDBIRTH

With scheduled surgical delivery dates and some foreknowledge of the cesarean delivery process, most (13; 81%) mothers focused on newborn health as their greatest labor and delivery concern. In fact, Ana was the only mother to mention any worry for her own well-being, saying, "They're afraid … [my placenta] may have attached itself to other organs, I think they were saying maybe my bladder." (Ana was most likely referring to the possibility of *placenta percreta*, a rare condition in which the uterus attaches so deeply that it penetrates through uterine tissue and attaches to another organ, such as the bladder. Placental abnormalities such as this occur more commonly among women who have previously had cesarean delivery; see Cunningham et al., 2009.)

With regard to fetal and newborn well-being, some mothers' concerns were general, as was Carolyn's worry about "something being wrong with the baby." Debra, who had been given news of "low amniotic fluid," spoke of staying healthy throughout pregnancy for her fetus's sake. Other mothers mentioned more specific concerns related to fetal and newborn health. For example, with premature birth a clear risk for her twins, Tasha worried most that "they might come premature," causing "complications" that could necessitate a long hospital stay. Mei, who already had a child with developmental disabilities, said she worried "all the time" about her next child's developing similar problems. Overall, however, unless mothers had cause for a specific concern, most described their chief worry in terms similar to Sharon's: "I'm not really all that uptight about any part of it … The health of the baby is of the utmost in my mind, and that's all I'm really concerned about."

Summary of Expectations and Fears in Mothers Planning Cesarean Delivery

The 16 mothers in this group did not share any single expectation, but the majority expected no experience of labor, whereas one mother suspected she might go into labor prematurely and another fully anticipated natural labor onset. Some but not all mothers reported expecting a short time from surgery to delivery, particularly if they had previously experienced labored cesarean. Other less frequently mentioned expectations included a long wait for surgery, pain, and negotiating newborn access with family members. Some mothers explicitly stated that they held no expectations. Perhaps because planned cesarean comprises a series of predetermined obstetric procedures, no mother in this group mentioned expectations related to receiving pain medication, fetal monitoring, maternal monitoring, or obstetric interventions apart from surgery itself. In discussing their childbirth-related fears, only one mother focused on her own well-being in childbirth, whereas nearly all mothers mentioned concerns related to fetal and newborn well-being. In some cases, concerns were general and in others, concerns related specifically to mothers' pregnancy status or previous births. Though most mothers mentioned fetal or newborn health as a chief or sole concern, no mother raised any particular concerns about possible negative consequences of cesarean birth for her newborn(s), including issues related to a shortened gestational period.

Confirmed and Violated Expectations in Planned Cesarean Birth

Fourteen of this chapter's mothers expected planned cesarean delivery with no labor onset, and that expectation was confirmed for 12 (86%). Six (38%) mothers experienced unanticipated changes to their surgical dates, and for all of these six, surgery advanced by a week or more than had been originally scheduled in order to prevent natural labor onset. One mother's suspicion that she might experience premature natural labor onset was confirmed. Three mothers had labored cesareans, but two of those had anticipated avoiding labor with planned cesarean. Four mothers experienced individual expectancy violations, including the violated expectation of a short wait time until delivery, the violated expectation of blocked sensation during surgery, and the violated expectation of natural labor onset.

Adding violations of the expectation to avoid labor to other individual expectancy violations, six (38%) mothers' childbirth expectations were violated, leaving ten (62%) mothers whose general expectations were confirmed. The experiences of all ten mothers who saw expectations generally confirmed involved some unanticipated event, such as a changed surgery date (in all cases, advanced), newborn health concerns, and others detailed later in individual case descriptions. In two instances, mothers viewed the unanticipated events and their overall experiences positively, and in the remaining cases, mothers reported negative responses or distress that did not always directly relate to the unanticipated events themselves.

Confirmed Expectations in Planned Cesarean Birth

Among mothers whose experiences generally confirmed expectations, Ana gave the most unequivocally positive report, beginning by saying that her overall experience "actually went beyond" her expectations. Her repeat cesarean surgery date was advanced by a week, a development that apparently caused her no concern. Hers was the first surgical appointment of the day, and at the appointed time, Ana walked herself into the operating room; this, in her words, was "kind of [the] hard part." She said the room was stocked with "extra blood and stuff," which she found unsettling in light of concerns her physician had raised about placental problems in pregnancy, but her surgery proceeded quickly and smoothly, and within two hours, Ana had her baby. Ana said, "The whole process … was just so scheduled out and so easy, and then they [say],

'OK, walk into the operating room'; it was just like wham, bam it was done; it was great … no problem at all." In the context of her heightened awareness of and likely associated fear about placental problems that did not develop, Ana's positive report seemed based largely on being relieved of that fear.

Sharon, also undergoing repeat cesarean surgery, said the overall experience "went as expected," though she did encounter unanticipated institutional issues. After arriving at the hospital on schedule, Sharon learned that the physician performing her surgery "was confused" about her due date. The physician sent Sharon to "have an ultrasound" and "perhaps … an amnio" to ensure that her fetus was sufficiently developed for birth. "I was not happy," Sharon said, remembering that her amniocentesis in pregnancy had caused severe bleeding requiring hospitalization. "Luckily," she said, the ultrasound indicated low amniotic fluid, so instead of performing amniocentesis, "they went ahead and did the c-section, and everything was fine." In this case, "fine" seemed to relate to having escaped a day of hospital tests and a rescheduled surgical date.

Heather, giving birth for the first time and not holding a "lot of expectations," said much of her birth experience "happened exactly the way" she had anticipated, except that she didn't realize surgery had begun when it did:

> The first one was born and he cried. And I was like, oh, I just gave birth. I had no clue. They were just, you know, chatting … I felt more like they were moving me on the table … adjusting me … They were going in after my kids, and I didn't know it.

Although Heather's surgery went smoothly and her newborns arrived healthy, her postpartum challenges reflect the risks of cesarean delivery, planned or otherwise. She had only a few isolated episodes of successful breastfeeding and struggled to obtain hospital assistance when her newborns had problems latching on. Heather said breastfeeding challenges left her feeling "depressed" because "I couldn't do what I thought I should be able to do. It was a mess." After her discharge, Heather's depressed feelings worsened, largely (by her account) because she had to discontinue breastfeeding. In addition, Heather found it hard to "get going" once at home in the midst of dealing with the demands of caring for two newborns while recovering from abdominal surgery. Her obstetrician prescribed medication, and Heather said her depression had mostly resolved.

Tasha, another mother of twins and one of the two mothers who stood out for her expectation that labor would begin naturally before her scheduled surgery date, saw her expectation confirmed when she felt strong contractions about a month before her planned delivery. She reported to the hospital, and after telling Tasha she had "probably been in labor all day," staff performed a labored cesarean delivery within two hours. Despite the premature labor onset that had concerned her during pregnancy, Tasha described her experience positively, saying, "Once the epidural was in, it was really nice and quick." Tasha also found herself pleasantly surprised by the absence of newborn complications. Her twins did, however, remain hospitalized in the NICU for five days because they had been born prematurely; she described her twins' current health as "outstanding."

Expectation Violated by No Natural Labor Onset

For second-time mother Ivey, who had fully anticipated natural labor onset prior to scheduled surgery, the surgical date was advanced by a week at her physician's recommendation in order to prevent labor, and contrary to her expectations, no natural labor occurred. This caused Ivey little if any apparent distress. In fact, Ivey said that the sum of her experiences was "actually better" than she could have anticipated, partly because she felt little pain ("I could barely feel it") and because her obstetrician, whom she had met once prior to her surgery

> gave me kind of a free tummy tuckie … which was really nice of him … He took about four inches off of my stomach. I was very happy about that. He said, 'Well, we took it up for your husband a little bit…' Everything went well. I was able to feed the baby right away.

Though Ivey described her tummy tuck as “free,” she did receive a bill of “like $35,000,” which she said her public insurance thankfully paid in full. She also received a stern warning from her obstetrician to avoid pregnancy in the near future due to extensive uterine scarring and uterine tissue that had been made, in her words, “kind of thin” by the two cesareans. As well as her surgery went, Ivey said she had been seeing a counselor for postpartum mood problems, which she described as “not mopey, but angry” feelings that she labeled depression.

Expectancy Violation by Perceived Excessive Wait Time

Mei, who had stated during pregnancy that she expected her planned cesarean to “go fast,” found herself unpleasantly surprised by what became an almost 10-hour process. Finding the overall experience vastly different than what she expected, Mei said, “I really thought that it would be faster … my daughter was delivered via emergency c-section, and it seemed to be much faster.” She believed that because this surgery was scheduled, “they took more time … it was probably twice as long.” Mei was further surprised when, after delivery, her newborn was immediately taken to the NICU for treatment of “problems breathing,” which sounded consistent with reported neonatal complications in cesarean birth. However, Mei attributed neonatal problems to the medical order she had received to fast before surgery; she said, “I think he was hungry … when they tried to feed him he was having trouble with the sucking and the swallowing so they put him in the NICU.” Mei’s baby remained hospitalized until her discharge three days later; Mei described her baby’s overall health as very good.

Expectancy Violation by Ineffective Pain Relief

Carolyn, who had previously delivered by labored cesarean, experienced a series of unanticipated childbirth events beginning with placental problems—specifically, placenta previa—which her doctor told her had arisen from her previous cesarean. Carolyn’s condition caused severe bleeding requiring hospitalization six weeks before her scheduled surgical date and ended with a distressing surgical experience.

A few weeks after her initial hospitalization, heavy bleeding began again, and Carolyn's obstetrician offered her the option of remaining hospitalized until her scheduled surgical date or undergoing cesarean delivery early. Carolyn agreed to surgery the next day. After "spinal" analgesia had been administered, surgery began, and Carolyn said that although she could "feel a whole lot," her request for additional medication was denied, leaving her "very uncomfortable," and aware of "everything that they were doing ... they were pulling him out, I could feel that pressure ... I could tell when she was sewing me back up, I could tell when she was sewing my uterus, my skin." Carolyn's baby had arrived four weeks early and "at first, had trouble breathing," so she was immediately taken to the NICU, where she remained until Carolyn's discharge three days later. Carolyn described her baby as "very healthy" today.

Expectancy Violation with Labored Cesarean

Gemma and Debra had labored cesareans, but neither mother went into labor before a scheduled surgical date. Rather, obstetric care and institutional issues resulted in both mothers' never having surgical dates firmly scheduled. Gemma, who during pregnancy understood her physician to say she would have a scheduled cesarean, said no further talk of planning cesarean delivery arose in subsequent prenatal visits, and she generously laughed when she said her overall experience had deviated from her expectations "by far." Natural labor began six days past her due date, and she went to the hospital, where she said staff told her she would "have the baby natural." After hospital labor of 15 hours with little progress, Gemma said, "Finally, they're all, 'Nope, we're doing an emergency c-section...' The doctor just decided. My skin was just too tight for him to even squish out of, I guess." Despite the unanticipated twists and turns on her pathway to delivery, Gemma cast her responses to it all in positive terms, saying things went, "Way easier ... way better than I expected. I didn't really feel that much pain."

Like Gemma's, Debra's violation of an expected planned cesarean resulted from complications with obstetric care itself, though (unlike Gemma) Debra had little positive to say about it. Anticipating the need for her parents' help with her older children postpartum, Debra traveled with her children across several states to her parents' home about two weeks before her scheduled surgery. Believing it would be difficult to find a doctor who would see a publicly insured patient in late pregnancy, Debra waited for natural labor onset and reported to the emergency department about two hours after labor began, where staff placed her in a waiting room, and a few hours later, "decided to do a c-section" as a matter of "hospital policy." Debra said,

> The doctors just seemed to be really uptight … They were angry with me for making the decision to have the baby back there when I hadn't even gotten my full maternity care there with one of their doctors … they said personal things about me with other doctors while they were doing my c-section—it was just [that] they didn't have any respect for me.

After her surgery, Debra said, the hospital obstetrician made her wait 24 hours to eat, which Debra believed interfered with her ability to produce sufficient milk for breastfeeding. Staff bottle-fed her baby with formula and were unavailable when she requested breastfeeding assistance. Shortly after hospital discharge, Debra stopped breastfeeding and switched to formula feeding.

Satisfaction

Hearing the majority of this chapter's mothers report feeling generally satisfied with planned surgeries that more often than not included advanced delivery schedules, maternal or neonatal complications, or institutional inefficiencies reminded me of Williams's (1994) statement that "satisfaction" with medical care may simply indicate relief that nothing extremely bad happened. For each of these mothers, "extremely bad" could be equated with the greatest childbirth fears they revealed during pregnancy. For example, Ana, who in pregnancy reported placental problems among her greatest fears and was reminded of those fears upon reporting to a delivery room stocked with "extra blood and stuff," had an uncomplicated surgical delivery process lasting less than two hours. Within that context, her unqualified report of feeling "very satisfied" could, as much as anything else, signify relief that the procedure went smoothly and nothing terrible happened. Similarly, Tasha, whose early and natural labor onset tested her fear of prematurely delivering her twins, was relieved of those fears when her newborns arrived in good health. Like Ana's, Tasha's surgery occurred within hours of her arrival at the hospital, and she found staff helpful and accommodating—all of which could be viewed as bonuses to the general relief of having passed an anticipated trouble spot. For Sharon, who nearly had to undergo an unanticipated amniocentesis as a condition of entering surgery as scheduled and instead unexpectedly underwent ultrasound, the relief at not having to endure the procedure she found objectionable and of not having to postpone surgery could easily have felt satisfactory compared to what might have come to pass.

For mothers whose expectations were violated, complex circumstances surrounding childbirth may have led them to equate "satisfaction" with their own and their offspring's arrival at the end of a long and tortuous road. For example, Carolyn faced late pregnancy hospitalization associated with her previous cesarean; in addition, her surgical dates were shifted, her expectation of effective pain treatment was violated, and her newborn was hospitalized. Yet as if in response to her own and her newborn's having survived all that, Carolyn reported feeling "very satisfied" overall, adding, "They immediately addressed [the newborn's] grunting and took her off right away … I felt like they really knew what they were doing and they did it well." Like Carolyn, Gemma had a birth experience that followed a circuitous (albeit different) path; her expectation of planned cesarean was violated because it was never scheduled. She went into labor naturally, and the experience concluded with labored cesarean. Despite this, Gemma said, "I'm satisfied—I'd go back!" She did, however, follow that with reference to perhaps more pressing worries related to covering mounting medical bills with no insurance or income.

Though surviving what in some cases sounded like aberrant birth experiences may have been sufficient for some women to report childbirth satisfaction, satisfaction was not in all cases unqualified, particularly when mothers felt they had received poor-quality care. For example, Heather changed her initial statement of feeling "really satisfied" with the experience of surgeons moving her on the table and "going in after [her] kids" to "not satisfied" when describing the "breastfeeding part," saying she wished she had received more help while in the hospital. Debra, who described enduring a surgery with a physician who spoke negatively of her throughout, directly referenced that behavior and the lack of postpartum breastfeeding support as the downsides to an otherwise "wonderful" experience. Whether Mei perceived as poor-quality care her long wait for her scheduled c-section or her newborn's being hospitalized immediately after delivery for what she believed was hunger, she stood out among this chapter's mothers in expressing an overwhelmingly negative view, saying, "The only good thing about it was having him afterwards, but this whole experience—I can't think of a single good thing about it."

Finally, Ivey's statement of general satisfaction with her planned cesarean surgery stands as a reminder of the dangers of relying solely on satisfaction reports as indicators of mothers' overall postpartum well-being. Ivey's birth experience involved a most unusual expectancy violation in the form of a "free tummy tuckie" (though with a $35,000 bill, perhaps *unexpected* would have been a more accurate word choice than *free*). Ivey reported feeling "extremely" satisfied, adding, "It was a very good experience." Setting aside my personal feelings about cosmetic surgery and a physician's reported decision to perform it on a woman for her husband's enjoyment, I found this mother's account of receiving surgery she had neither requested nor anticipated most troubling because the physician behavior Ivey described—performing an unnecessary procedure unrelated to her obstetric needs—violated hard-won patients' rights to informed consent. On the one hand, fortunately (and improbably) the seemingly nonconsensual tummy tuck caused Ivey no immediate adverse physical or financial consequences. On the other hand, Ivey's enthusiasm over the procedure and her "extreme" satisfaction conflicted with the later postpartum mood problems she reported, which seemed more consistent with the sum of her childbirth experiences, including scheduling a cesarean with virtually no maternal input into the decision (alongside her apparent gross misunderstanding of her own medical rights), advancing the surgical date, and receiving an unexpected procedure on the surgical table.

Summary and Implications

Cesarean delivery may be planned well in advance of a mother's due date on the premise that the risk of natural labor outweighs the risks of surgery, and arriving at that decision appears, increasingly, to involve professional and institutional preference as much as or even more than clear scientific evidence. It is almost understood that among available contemporary birth approaches, planned cesarean reigns as the most technocratically oriented because its execution relies primarily on physicians and medical technology, and the mother's role is largely restricted to appearing at the appointed place and time for surgery. Most of this study's mothers were pursuing planned cesarean delivery as repeat procedures following a previous cesarean without any other identified medical indication. The role of physician input into mothers' ultimate decisions to pursue planned cesarean delivery varied case by case, though not a single mother reported that her physician had discussed the balance of surgical risks versus labor risks or nonsurgical birth alternatives. With that seemingly narrow view as the backdrop for their upcoming births, these mothers' expectations reflected a limited maternal role in surgical birth, with most focusing on the aspects of the experience that planned cesarean delivery is designed to control, such as avoiding labor or having a predicable labor-to-delivery wait time.

In terms of what mothers can expect in the contemporary United States' technocratic birth culture, planned cesarean delivery, at least on the surface, seems to offer the greatest promise of expectancy confirmation because this approach narrows the scope of possibility for either maternal interests or maternal physiology to run counter to its design. Planning cesarean delivery implies acceptance of a standard obstetric treatment package, greatly reducing the chances that any unexpected intervention may become part of a mother's birth experience. Moreover, the planned cesarean delivery package eliminates maternal guesswork on physical aspects of the normal labor process, such as when labor might begin (most assume it will not), how long it might last (most expect a short surgery-to-delivery time line), and when and how the newborn will arrive (by cesarean on the date of surgery).

With numerous possible expectations addressed in advance, the probability of violated expectations would seem to be correspondingly reduced. As evidence supporting that supposition, the 62% rate of expectancy confirmation among this chapter's mothers ranked highest among all other hospital-birthing groups (the planned epidural group came in a close second, at 59%). Although 10 mothers' experiences met their general expectations, such as avoiding labor, each of those 10 also described some unanticipated labor and delivery event. In two cases, mothers described unanticipated events in the context of an otherwise positive experience with no mention of negative feelings: Ana reported having had her surgical date advanced by a week and having her surgery proceed even more smoothly than she could have imagined; relieved of concerns that her placenta might have attached to her internal organs, Ana's report contained no mention of negative responses except feeling shaken by walking herself into surgical quarters. Tasha, whose twins' premature arrival partly confirmed her worries, nevertheless described her overall experience and responses with a noteworthy absence of negativity. Attached to both Ana's and Tasha's positive reports were the two mothers' references to institutional efficiency—in Ana's words, "wham, bam, it was done," and in Tasha's, the process was "really nice and quick."

Along with maternal expectations of technological birth come expectations of greater childbirth efficiency than old-fashioned labor and vaginal delivery. A number of mothers undergoing repeat cesarean said as much in expressing expectations of a smoother birth experience than their previous labored cesarean experience or a short labor-to-delivery time line. Ana's and Tasha's positive reports of their experiences only underscored that expectation. To consistently fulfill such an expectation, however, institutions offering planned cesarean birth must consistently maintain organizational efficiency, ensuring that adequate and communicative staff are available to perform the surgery and to address the full range of consequences it imposes. When institutions fall short on those measures, the risk of unexpected distress rises even among mothers whose surgical process might have gone smoothly and whose expectations were otherwise confirmed.

For example, Sharon experienced apparent institutional inefficiency when her physician reportedly could not clearly discern her due date, obliging her to undergo additional obstetric procedures, to which she naturally responded negatively. Heather, whose birth otherwise confirmed expectations, referred negatively to the hospital staff's unresponsiveness to her requests for help breastfeeding, even connecting her postpartum distress to problems she believed stemmed from inadequate professional attention. Debra, who also reported poor staff response to requested breastfeeding assistance, saw her birth expectations violated in numerous ways but attached her negative feelings as much to inadequate breastfeeding help as to unanticipated negativity from her surgeons. As one final example, Mei, who waited long hours in the hospital for her scheduled surgery, described her planned cesarean delivery in wholly negative terms, saying she could not think of a "single good thing" about the overall experience.

When the economic bottom line constantly looms, as it does in contemporary U.S. health care at large, an explicit or implicit expectation of an efficient planned cesarean birth experience with fully supported follow-up care greatly risks violation. Moreover, these mothers' accounts remind one that expectation of planned cesarean birth free of its established risks is at equal or even greater risk of violation. For example, one mother (Carolyn) experienced placenta previa, one had vaguely stated placental issues (Ana), and another (Ivey) was warned against becoming pregnant again too soon because of her uterine condition, all of which are established risks associated with cesarean surgery. Three mothers' newborns were hospitalized in the NICU immediately postpartum, and two others reported problems breastfeeding. These cesarean-related consequences occurred across mothers who did and did not have their expectations generally confirmed, but perhaps more concerning was how few had mentioned any anticipation that these known cesarean risks might become part of their stories.

At best, planned cesarean delivery can offer an efficient and adequately supported experience to help mothers recover smoothly and ease into their anticipated role, which many define by the ability to breastfeed. Just two of this chapter's 16 mothers gave accounts of planned cesarean delivery "at its best," describing smooth, uncomplicated surgeries free of institutional delays, professional misbehavior, or other complications. And for these women, cesarean delivery "at its best" meant getting through the experience without having their worst fears confirmed. But a more realistic picture of planned cesarean birth should include the sorts of unanticipated events reported by most of this chapter's mothers, including shifting surgical schedules, poor follow-up care, and even professional violations of ethical codes on informed consent. Such events highlight what more generally characterizes this chapter's maternal accounts: one or more instances of a negative professional, institutional, or medical consequence directly related to the surgery itself.

This chapter's mothers spoke of general satisfaction in the face of what sounded like aversive childbirth experiences, a fact that I believe attests their overall relief at having avoided something potentially even more nightmarish. Mothers like Carolyn, who had placenta previa and an NICU-hospitalized newborn, said, "Things don't always go as you planned … It's not that bad … [and] you recover. If that's what they have to do, that's what needs to be done. Am I devastated by it? No." As gracefully as Carolyn weathered her experience, it would be unfair for anyone to expect all mothers to endure negative birth events with similar resilience, particularly when such events could have been prevented with better quality care and decision making focused on long-term maternal health.

ENDNOTE

1. The question of an "ideal" cesarean rate was addressed in a seminal World Health Organization–sponsored study of widely varying cesarean delivery rates (1–80%) across Latin American countries. Cesarean rates of 1–5% corresponded to high maternal and neonatal mortality and serious complications, but those problems declined steadily as the cesarean rate climbed toward 15%. However, once surgical rates exceeded 15%, they were accompanied by concomitant increases in mortality and serious complications (Villar, Valladares, & Wojdyla, 2006). The 15% rate, less than half the early 21st-century U.S. rate of 32%, exists as a guideline; arguably, the safest approach is consistently providing mothers the best available care in light of their individual circumstances.

Chapter 7

Expectations and Experiences of Vaginal Birth after Cesarean (VBAC)

The Context of VBAC

In reference to planned cesarean delivery meant to circumvent the strain of labor on previous cesarean surgical scars, the American College of Obstetricians and Gynecologists employed the phrase *elective repeat cesarean delivery*, or ERCD (e.g., ACOG, 2010, 2011a). Some have proposed that the term *elective* inaccurately implies a lack of medical rationale (Berghella, Blackwell, Ramin, Sibai, & Saade, 2011). Although I would agree that *elective* is imprecise, as evidenced in chapter 6's maternal reports of physician and other external influences on their repeat cesarean decisions, the term calls attention to two facts: First, more than 90% of mothers who have previously delivered by cesarean have ERCD in subsequent births in the absence of any other medical risk

(Menacker & Hamilton, 2010). Second, the descriptor *elective* in repeat cesarean delivery reminds one that cesarean is an alternative to what in most cases is an equally viable option, vaginal birth. However, precisely how viable vaginal birth after cesarean (VBAC) is and how that in turn influences maternal expectations warrant discussion.

First, I wish to clarify a few terms. Though a mother may plan on VBAC, planned VBAC results in vaginal birth in 60–80% of cases (e.g., Cunningham et al., 2010; Menacker & Hamilton, 2010). Reflecting the two possible outcomes of planned VBAC, the expression *trial of labor after cesarean* (TOLAC) is used; "successful" TOLAC refers to vaginal delivery and "unsuccessful" TOLAC, to labored cesarean. Because the phrase *trial of labor* immediately brings to mind the possibility of cesarean delivery, I instead use *planned VBAC*, emphasizing the preferred childbirth pathway. To encompass the variety of influences on mothers' decisions to pursue "elective" repeat cesarean delivery (see chapter 6), I instead use *planned repeat cesarean delivery* (PRCD).

Planned VBAC comes with the usual risks of vaginal delivery, including the worrisome yet remote possibility of uterine rupture. However, as cesarean rates began rising in the 1960s and surgical techniques correspondingly advanced, a National Institutes of Health (NIH) expert panel concluded, based on available evidence, that VBAC was safe (NIH, 1981). Subsequently, VBAC rates began ticking steadily upward, nearly doubling from 3.4% in 1980 to 6.6% in 1985 (Taffel, Placek, Moien, & Kosary, 1991) and reaching an all-time high of 28.3% of postcesarean births in 1996 (Martin et al., 2006). The VBAC upswing was matched by corresponding drops in the overall U.S. cesarean delivery rate, which dipped to 20.7% in 1996 (Martin et al., 2006).

However, VBAC rates began a steady retreat starting in 1996, the same year a *New England Journal of Medicine* publication reported outcomes on over 6,000 Canadian women giving birth after previous cesarean: Neonatal outcomes did not differ between VBAC and PRCD groups, but uterine rupture and emergency hysterectomy were reported 1.8 times more frequently in VBAC mothers (McMahon, Luther, Bowes, & Olshan, 1996). That report came amidst rising rates of vaginal birth interventions designed to intensify uterine activity—namely, artificial labor induction and acceleration with medications. Increased uterine activity heightens the risk of uterine rupture, and in response to evidence of this, ACOG published a statement in 1999 advising hospitals against performing VBAC without specific preparations, such as having an "immediately available" anesthesiologist to support emergency cesarean. Since ACOG's 1999 publication, VBAC rates have steadily declined, and as of 2007, the VBAC rate hovered around 8%, with all indications pointing to a continuing downward trend (Menacker & Hamilton, 2010).

ACOG's 1999 policy has been pointed to as one of the strongest forces—if not the primary force—behind the reversal in the late 20th-century U.S. VBAC trend. Specifically, ACOG's restrictive institutional preparedness recommendations led some hospitals to enact VBAC bans, claiming resource shortages as insurmountable barriers. In an example of the ACOG policy's chilling effect, of 300 hospitals, one third of those that had previously offered VBAC stopped doing so after the release of ACOG's 1999 guidelines; of hospitals that continued to offer VBAC, 68% instituted more restrictive policies (Roberts, Deutchman, King, Fryer, & Miyoshi, 2007). Hospitals offering VBAC tend to be larger, to be located in urban centers, and to process more patients—further restricting access to VBAC for women in specific areas. Other institutions simply disallow VBAC without any expressed policy (de facto bans); some insurance companies have followed suit by reimbursing repeat cesarean but not VBAC births.

In a move similar to the NIH's response to cesarean rate increases in the 21st century, the NIH has again assembled an expert panel to address VBAC issues. A panel review of over 900 published studies on planned VBAC found that despite being generally low, maternal mortality was almost four times higher in women undergoing PRCD than in those undergoing planned VBAC, with death rates of 13.4 and 3.8 per 100,000, respectively. Other serious outcomes, including hysterectomy, hemorrhage, and blood transfusions were similar for both planned VBAC and PRCD (Guise et al., 2010). Uterine rupture was higher in VBAC, with a reported 4.7 events per 1,000, compared to 0.3 per 1,000 in PRCD; 7% of all rupture cases were associated with perinatal death (stillbirth or newborn death within one week after birth; WHO, 2006). A subsequent multidisciplinary NIH consensus development panel reinforced those findings, reporting that higher maternal mortality, longer hospitalization, more placental problems in later pregnancies, and more serious blood clot events in PRCD make VBAC generally the safer option for mothers (Cunningham et al., 2010).

Both 21st-century NIH VBAC review panels highlighted difficulties in assessing outcomes because existing studies often collapse "successful" and "unsuccessful" planned VBACs into one group that is then compared to PRCD, precluding full confidence in the state of current scientific knowledge. Rozen, Ugoni, and Sheehan (2011) took that notion a step further, proposing that a more appropriate comparison group for women planning VBAC would be other women planning vaginal birth without previous cesarean delivery. In a review of over 21,000 mothers' medical records, the authors found no differences on maternal or neonatal outcomes between first-time mothers delivering vaginally and VBAC mothers, excepting a slightly higher rate of shoulder dystocia and instrumental delivery in the VBAC group.

With the complexity surrounding tradeoffs between both the remote and more commonly occurring relative risks of planned VBAC and PRCD, childbirth professionals and interest groups have raised concern about the influence of medicolegal liability in professional medical organizations' policies and related restrictions on maternal VBAC and cesarean delivery options (cf. Fuglenes, Oian, & Kristiansen, 2009). For example, contained in an NIH 2010 VBAC consensus panel statement was this quotation: "The panel is concerned that medical-legal considerations add to, and in many instances exacerbate, these [professional] barriers to trial of labor" (Cunningham et al., 2010, p. 3). A related editorial emphasized that the professional obstetric community should evaluate how medical guidelines based largely on litigation concerns affect the maternal medical decision-making process (Shorten, 2010). Demonstrating potential nonscientific influences on VBAC guidelines, an analysis of VBAC guidelines from six English speaking nations found that all relied heavily on clinical consensus and scientific data of low quality or with inconclusive results (Foureur, Ryan, Nicholl, & Homer, 2010).

In response to climbing repeat cesarean delivery rates and related criticisms regarding its role in the situation, ACOG issued a slightly less restrictive VBAC policy in 2010. Discussing its 1999 recommendation that certain hospital services be "immediately available," ACOG wrote, "Although there is reason to think that more rapid availability of cesarean delivery may provide a small incremental benefit in safety, comparative data examining in detail the effect of alternate systems and response times are not available" (ACOG, 2010, p. 457). ACOG did, however, remain firm in its recommendation that physicians "uncomfortable" with a patient's interest in pursuing VBAC should refer such patients to another provider (ACOG, 2011a). However, finding a willing VBAC provider is likely to become increasingly difficult: A 2009 ACOG practitioner survey found that more than 60% of obstetricians reported making liability-related practice changes, with 29.1% reporting that they increased their cesarean delivery rate and 29.5% reporting that they had ceased overseeing VBACs.

Retired obstetrician Perl (2010) reflected that medical professionals currently in training see PRCD and the current 30% (and up) cesarean rate as normal, failing to question the medical indications of repeat cesarean surgery or to consider maternal thoughts on the matter. In terms of what mothers think, the few available studies on mothers' decisions about and expectations of VBAC—none of which was conducted in the United States—generally underscore a strong personal commitment to VBAC on the belief that natural birth is better for mother and baby. Positive VBAC reports from friends and family often influenced mothers' decisions to plan VBAC, and many mothers found that extensive efforts, such as changing physicians or hospitals, obtaining second opinions, and restating their VBAC interests, were required to secure the approach (Fenwick, Gamble, & Hauck, 2007; Meddings, Phipps, Haith-Cooper, & Haigh, 2007; Phillips, McGrath, & Vaughan, 2009–2010).

With the early 21st-century United States' massive culture change in VBAC practitioner and institutional availability, mothers desiring the approach may indeed find themselves having to aggressively pursue it. The International Cesarean Awareness Network (I-CAN), exists to educate women on their VBAC rights and to help them find VBAC birth attendants and resources.

STUDY MOTHERS ANTICIPATING VBAC

Of this study's 75 total mothers, five (7%) were planning VBAC. All five were having second children subsequent to a first birth that had concluded in labored or emergency cesarean. Mothers' education ranged from high school to bachelor's degree; family income ranged from slightly above poverty to middle income. All five mothers were younger than age 31. One mother was nonwhite. All had private health insurance. All five VBAC mothers were married or had stable partners, and all mothers in this group stayed at home full time. Following the approach outlined in chapter 1, I discuss findings for the whole group, providing quotations and examples of experiences drawn from select representative cases; mothers' names are fictional.

Four of this group's five mothers voiced a personal commitment to vaginal birth that predated their first birth and cesarean delivery. Annette said, "I wanted to have a natural birth, had planned to all along." Along similar lines, she said she thought contemporary obstetric intervention was generally "over the top" and that she wanted to be "in control" of medical decisions and the interventions she received.

Common among the five VBAC mothers and similar to most later-time mothers in this text, all five mothers planning VBAC spoke to how their previous births had influenced their VBAC decisions. For most in this chapter, the previous cesarean delivery experience had been negative, and their VBAC decisions came partly in response to, and were even intensified as a result of, previous emergency cesarean deliveries that they described in terms suggestive of trauma. As examples, both Annette and Natalie described their previous cesarean births as having been performed shortly after hospital admission, under general anesthesia, and without their full awareness or understanding of what was occurring. In Annette's case, staff discovered shortly after her arrival at the hospital that her fetus was in breech position; she was "knocked out right away" and "didn't even know what was going on." She continued, "I didn't get to breastfeed right away … I was disappointed … about not having even been awake … it was so long afterwards to even be able to hold the baby." Along similar lines, Natalie said that she had fully expected and looked forward to natural birth in the hospital. Once she arrived there in labor, however, she said she had "absolutely no control over" what happened next. Natalie said staff "suddenly freaked out," and before she knew it, she was "completely knocked out"; her newborn arrived later by cesarean.

Marta, whose previous cesarean had been performed to address fetal heart-rate concerns after several hours of hospital labor, cast her cesarean experience in a mostly positive light, saying, "I felt basically no pain. You know, I had great pain relief." Attributing her largely positive experience to her physician's care, she had gone to great lengths to secure the same obstetrician's services for her upcoming birth. Recalling a long and difficult recovery from her first cesarean, Marta reacted to her physician's statement that she would have a "decent chance" of successful VBAC with "I'd rather have that [VBAC] for the sake of recovery than [be] cut open."

In discussing their pursuit of VBAC, all mothers except Marta made some reference to having received the message that they were making a relatively unusual decision. For example, Annette said that after she made her VBAC plan known to her physician, he reminded her that she could plan cesarean "right off the bat" and provided extensive warnings about "stuff that could happen." As she stood firm on her VBAC decision, she said, "They had us sign some paperwork that that is what we had discussed." Already somewhat aware of VBAC's relative rarity, Natalie said the lack of willing VBAC providers in her large metropolitan area reminded her of just how rare her decision was; she eventually found an obstetrician through I-CAN.

EXPECTATIONS IN MOTHERS PLANNING VBAC

All mothers in this group expected to have vaginal delivery in a hospital; Marta was the only one to mention the possibility of cesarean delivery, which she said she would "automatically" have if she passed her due date because of her physician's concerns about an "old placenta." All mothers referred to expecting childbirth pain. Until prompted, mothers did not mention expectations related to specific obstetric procedures, such as labor induction, fetal monitoring, labor acceleration, medical pain relief, or episiotomy. When prompted, all mothers indicated an expectation of electronic fetal monitoring based on previous experience. However, mothers generally did not expect to have other interventions; only Natalie said she did not expect to have an epidural but "wasn't sure" because she had not "had normal labor" before. Marta spoke of being unsure whether to expect most interventions, saying she fully trusted her physician "to make the best decisions" about what might or might not be become necessary during labor.

Among less frequently mentioned expectations were three mothers' expectations of having a less stressful birth experience than previous experiences, particularly because their first births had been treated as medical emergencies or had involved maternal notification of a problematic fetal health issue. Two mothers mentioned expectations of participating more in the birth process than they had previously. Annette compared that expectation to her feeling of being "robbed" of a normal birth experience the first time around, which she described as something that was "just done" to her. Along with her expectation of participating more in childbirth this time, Natalie said she looked forward to "seeing what" her body "could do" without extensive medical assistance or intervention.

Though she had expected vaginal delivery, Annette stood out as the only mother in this group to say she believed "anything could happen" in the context of her childbirth expectation. Perhaps because cesarean delivery had occurred within hours of their arrival at the hospital in their previous births, no mothers in this group mentioned expectations related to labor duration. No one mentioned expecting vaginal birth or VBAC complications for themselves or their newborns.

Greatest Fears in Childbirth

All VBAC mothers ranked repeat cesarean delivery as their top if not only childbirth concern. For example, Natalie worried most that her upcoming birth would involve "cesarean, medical interventions ... an emergency that I have no control over." Annette and Natalie also worried about repeat cesarean surgery's becoming necessary, but they qualified their statements with reference to some advantage present in their current situation. Annette had been receiving frequent ultrasounds because of concerns about cervical dilation, so she believed she would receive notice of a necessary repeat cesarean well in advance, making it less of "an emergency." Marta said that her trust in her physician helped reduce her worries about possible cesarean, and that her greater concern was that a repeat cesarean would be a less positive experience than her first, saying, "I would want it to be as good as it happened with the first. I probably should prepare myself that it won't."

Summary of VBAC Mothers' Expectations and Fears

Mothers planning VBAC all expected hospital birth, and though all expected vaginal delivery, one mother mentioned her awareness that her VBAC plan could change to PRCD if she were to pass her due date before going into labor naturally. All mothers expected childbirth pain, and they all expected electronic fetal monitoring based on their previous birth experiences. Mothers either did not expect or expressed uncertainty about other birth interventions, such as labor induction, labor acceleration, and episiotomy. No mother referred to expecting specific VBAC or vaginal birth consequences. All mothers referred to cesarean delivery as the chief childbirth concern, with one mother narrowing the focus of her concern to a potential repeat cesarean experience that would be less satisfactory than her previous one.

CONFIRMED AND VIOLATED EXPECTATIONS IN MOTHERS PLANNING VBAC

Of this chapter's five mothers, two (40%) experienced VBAC as they had anticipated. Both mothers delivering by VBAC went into labor naturally (no induction). For one of those two, amniotomy was her only reported birth intervention, and the other mentioned having received a local anesthetic injection before her physician stitched up a minor perineal tear. Two (40%) mothers had their expectations of vaginal birth violated by switches from VBAC to planned repeat cesarean (PRCD) in their final weeks of pregnancy. Both PRCD cases involved physician recommendation related to concerns about continuing pregnancy as due dates approached (reflected in Marta's case, described later). One mother's vaginal birth expectation was violated by labored cesarean delivery involving multiple interventions.

Case of Confirmed Expectation of VBAC

Annette, whose first breech birth had concluded in an emergency cesarean delivery for which she reported being "knocked out" and of which she became aware only hours later, had her expectations and related desire for VBAC fully confirmed. Annette described her total 14-hour labor as beginning at about 3:00 a.m. the day before her due date. Because her "contractions weren't bad," Annette said, she worked in her yard on and off the next morning, then remembered to call the hospital because she had experienced a short first labor, and "they said come right in." Annette reported to the hospital around noon, settled into a room, and about four hours passed without her labor's progressing "a whole lot." To help move things along, Annette said, "they broke my water and within 45 minutes the baby was born. Everything went as well as I could have expected, even better. I'm just ecstatic that I was able to do it."

Case of Violated Expectation with Switch from Planned VBAC to Repeat Cesarean

During pregnancy, Marta had been aware that she would "automatically have" a cesarean delivery if she went past her due date. However,

VBAC that many women face, Annette said she had shared her VBAC story with friends who might someday find themselves in a similar position.

In contrast to mothers in other vaginal-birth groups whose expectations were somehow violated yet who reported moderate if not qualified satisfaction, this chapter's mothers with violated expectations reported low overall satisfaction with their experiences. For example, Natalie, who underwent labored cesarean rather than VBAC, reported feeling "not that satisfied." Natalie softened her statement by saying she felt good about not "automatically going for" repeat cesarean delivery, about having taken as active a role as she believed she could have in the labored cesarean delivery decision, and about having stood firm on her wishes for newborn hospital care, saying, "I think that if it had been up to them, I would have been a lot more unhappy. I was in control with little things that were happening … That was able to make it better."

Unlike Natalie, Marta focused less on her violated VBAC expectation as the source of her dissatisfaction and instead attached her lingering negative feelings about the entire experience to postoperative events, saying, "If this had been my first experience, I would have been horrified. I would have been like, oh my gosh, don't ever let me have any more kids … if I have to have c-sections." Marta assumed some undue responsibility for the postoperative care she received, at first reflecting on how she could have done "a better job" familiarizing herself with "aftercare of c-sections," but then added, "In this day and age … [considering] everything they know about pain relief … you really shouldn't be feeling like that in this country."

Summary and Implications

Changes in the historic obstetric professional maxim "once a cesarean, always a cesarean" began changing in the 20th century's later decades as improved cesarean surgical techniques led to greater safety in subsequent labor and vaginal birth, influencing a temporary, late 20th-century upswing in U.S. VBAC rates and a corresponding decrease in cesarean birth. However, complex forces, including rare though documented VBAC risks, increasing obstetric practices potentially intensifying those risks, and professional and hospital policy sensitive to medicolegal liability risk have resulted in shrinking VBAC availability and practice. In describing their decisions to pursue VBAC, several of this study's five mothers planning VBAC described having dealt with documented VBAC barriers.

Of the five mothers in this group, three underwent TOLAC, and two of those cases concluded in vaginal delivery. This study's 67% TOLAC vaginal birth "success" rate paralleled a national report of 60–80% "success" (e.g., Cunningham et al., 2010; Menacker & Hamilton, 2010). The other two of this group's five mothers originally expressed anticipation of VBAC but changed their plans to repeat cesarean delivery in the final weeks of pregnancy in light of concerns their obstetric caregivers reportedly expressed as the mothers' due dates approached. Adding those two mothers to the three who actually underwent a trial of labor, the percentage of mothers whose experiences confirmed their original VBAC expectations dropped to 40% of all mothers in this group.

With two of five study mothers having switched from planned VBAC to PRCD in late pregnancy, a VBAC expectation or plan seems most appropriately defined as a dynamic and moving target. Moreover, the VBAC target appeared to move not entirely as a matter of medical risk. Rather, in the absence of clearly identified risk, mothers were presented with an even more restricted VBAC option than they originally had primarily as a function of physician availability as their newborns' arrival dates neared. Under the circumstances, use of the appellation *elective repeat cesarean delivery* seems all the more problematic because the culture at large—and some obstetric professionals, judging by the frequent and misleading references to "cesarean delivery on maternal request" that appear in medical publications—tends to view mothers as the ones electing the approach, though this is not accurate. Furthermore, the subject pool of mothers undergoing PRCD may be swelling with mothers originally deemed good candidates for VBAC, an important consideration for further research on VBAC and PRCD medical and psychological outcomes.

Though this group contained only five mothers, extensively interviewing them in late pregnancy and again postpartum contributed to the existing limited understanding of violated VBAC expectations. A VBAC expectation can be violated well before birth when the birth approach changes to PRCD. However, common among mothers whose VBAC expectations were violated by either planned or labored cesarean was reported dissatisfaction at having undergone cesarean, at the occurrence of an unanticipated event in postpartum hospitalization, or both. This finding was consistent with the one available non-U.S. study on effects of VBAC expectancy violations, a study that indicated high maternal frustration over repeat labored cesarean and concerns about being negatively judged for having "failed" at the attempt (McGrath, Phillips, & Vaughan, 2010). The uniformly low satisfaction reported by this study's mothers whose VBAC expectations were violated contrasted with satisfaction among mothers in other childbirth-approach groups, such as natural childbirth or planned cesarean, who often reported moderate to high, if not qualified, satisfaction.

Consistent with previous studies on women pursuing VBAC (e.g., Fenwick et al., 2007; Meddings et al., 2007; Phillips et al., 2009–2010), most mothers in this chapter reported pursuing VBAC based on an original commitment to natural childbirth that predated and was subsequently violated in their first births. In addition, with the exception of Marta, mothers in this group struggled to secure the VBAC option. When mothers renewed their vaginal birth expectation by planning VBAC only to experience a violation similar to their first, the cumulative effect must have certainly influenced their overall views on and satisfaction with the second births. And for this study's mothers in particular, the VBAC expectancy violation also confirmed what they reported as their greatest worries during pregnancy—as in, for example, Natalie's worry about having a second cesarean and Marta's about having a second cesarean that might go less smoothly than her first. In contrast, confirmation of one's VBAC plan with vaginal delivery in a second birth must seem like double victory, leading to the unequivocally positive feelings Annette, for one, reported about the experience.

An alternative or perhaps adjunct explanation for maternal dissatisfaction associated with violated VBAC expectations was the occurrence of unanticipated surgical follow-up-care events similar to those reported in chapter 6 among mothers who underwent planned cesarean birth and contributing to parallel negative feelings. Specifically, both Natalie and Marta attached their expressed dissatisfaction with the quality of care they received in postsurgical hospitalization, not unlike mothers in chapter 6 who found cesarean surgery itself satisfactory but were distressed by, for example, the lack of staff response to their postsurgical requests for assistance. The sum of these mothers' reports suggests that, consistent with the contemporary technocratic orientation towards obstetric care in the United States, "care" may be limited to effective performance of a technologically advanced surgical procedure, whereas nontechnical aspects of care, such as responding to "nonurgent" requests for pain relief or for help with newborn care, seem to rank lower in priority.

Most in the obstetric profession would say that the first emphasis of obstetric care is ensuring maternal and fetal survival and safety, requiring that priority dedication of energy and resources focus on maintaining top-notch technical performance of obstetric interventions, such as cesarean surgery. Most would also likely agree that superior technical performance should occur in an overall context of full and appropriate support for maternal and newborn needs, even those perceived as nonurgent. However, it should nevertheless be recognized that in the culture of profit-driven health care, advanced surgical techniques generate more institutional income than do timely professional responses to requests for follow-up care that are perceived as nonurgent. In fact, the latter may be more of an economic liability than asset in the overall contemporary health-care equation because providing such care may require expanding a lean, cost-efficient staff. In such an environment, mothers and professionals might do well to prepare themselves for the realistic possibility that nonsurgical care may fail to live up even to entirely reasonable maternal expectations.

Regardless of whether they experienced negative childbirth events or violated expectations, however, all this chapter's mothers made effortful attempts to draw their stories to a close on a positive note. This is not to imply that whatever happened to the mothers was necessarily acceptable or that having a healthy newborn somehow compensated for negative childbirth events. Instead, in the face of events that at times sounded far from acceptable, these mothers evidenced remarkable emotional resilience in attempting to salvage something good from a bad situation over which they had little control. For Annette, on the one hand, whose VBAC experience confirmed her expectations and went as smoothly as one could hope, concluding on a positive note seemed most natural. On the other hand, Marta had to look beyond her postoperative trauma to find any upside to her story, though she managed to do it: "The beginning was definitely worse ... But in the long run ... my recovery has been quicker." Natalie concluded her story by saying, "What are you going to do? It's taken some time to get over [it] and move on ... but it's OK."

Chapter 8

Expectations and Experiences of Out-of-Hospital Birth

The Context of Out-of-Hospital Birth

About a century ago, nearly 100% of U.S. women expected to give birth at home, but a steady, irreversible trend toward hospital birth began (see chapter 1); by 1969, the percentage of home births had bottomed out at 1%, and it has remained relatively stable since. Even with a slight early 21st-century uptick in U.S. out-of-hospital births, the percentage remains in the 1% range, with about one third of those occurring in freestanding birth centers (birth settings unconnected to hospitals) and the remaining two thirds in women's homes (MacDorman, Menacker, & Declercq, 2010). Washington and Oregon, the two states from which most of this book's interviewees were drawn, rank among the top 10 U.S. states in national home-birth rates. Because most out-of-hospital births occur in women's homes and because this chapter's mothers all had home births except one (who delivered in a birth center), the remainder of this discussion focuses primarily on home birth.

Critical to understanding the current debate surrounding home-birth safety and other outcomes is first the distinction between planned and unplanned home birth. In planned home birth, a mother consciously decides on and arranges for home birth well in advance. Similar to those planning VBAC (chapter 7), mothers planning home birth may have to take extensive steps—for example, identifying a trustworthy attendant and arranging finances. Despite an estimated cost savings of 68% in an "average" home birth compared to an uncomplicated hospital vaginal birth (R. E. Anderson & D. A. Anderson, 1999), public and private insurers alike may not reimburse any home-birth costs, reflecting a general professional and cultural bias favoring hospital birth. With data available only from the 19 states that track whether home births were planned or unplanned, planned home births constituted about 83% of U.S. home births in 2006, and this group of mothers consisted largely of women who had attended college, who were in their 30s or older, married, and white (Declercq, MacDorman, Menacker, & Stotland, 2010). The remaining 17% of early 21st-century U.S. home births were unplanned, defined as occurring spontaneously and for reasons that include premature labor, precipitous (fast) labor, and no connection to professional medical care. In 2006, unplanned home births tended to occur among women who were nonwhite, foreign-born, under age 30, and who had no prenatal care; unplanned home births also involved more preterm deliveries (Declercq et al., 2010).

Second in understanding home-birth safety and outcomes is identifying who attends the birth and what connections that person has to hospital obstetric services. In nations such as Canada, Britain, and the Netherlands, certified professional midwives attend nearly all home births (e.g., Janssen et al., 2002; U.K. Home Birth Reference Site, 2011; Wiegers, van der Zee, & Keirse, 1998), and because midwifery credentialing and practice are nationally regulated and midwives are full-fledged members of the health-care system, they continue participating in the mother's care if emergency hospital services become necessary. In contrast, at the time of this writing, the United States had no national policies on home-birth attendants, nor did national policies exist surrounding home-birth attendants' access to hospital services, so if a mother requires emergency hospital services, her birth attendant may or may not be involved beyond the point of hospital admission. In 2006, 61% of U.S. home births were attended by midwives (16% certified nurse-midwives, 45% "other" midwives, a group that could include professional midwives and those with no formal training), 7.6% by physicians, and the remaining 36% by "other" individuals, such as a family member, an emergency medical technician, or a taxi driver (Declercq et al., 2010).

Studies on home-birth outcomes generally share two features: (1) Mothers at some point prior to labor indicated a preference for birthing at home, and (2) a credentialed birth attendant, usually a professional midwife, assisted. When those criteria are met, data indicate that home-birthing mothers undergo significantly fewer obstetric interventions, but other maternal and neonatal outcomes appear similar. For example, a 21st-century North American study including over 5000 mothers intending to deliver at home (98% from the United States) showed rates of perinatal and neonatal mortality (stillbirth or death within 7 days postpartum, and newborn death within 28 days postpartum, respectively; WHO, 2006) comparable to those in a large low-risk, midwife-attended hospital comparison group (Johnson & Daviss, 2005). About 12% of home-birth mothers were transported to hospitals; labor induction rates were 9.6% in the home-birth group and 21% in the hospital comparison group; episiotomy rates were 2.1% and 33%, cesarean delivery rates were 3.7% and 19.0%, and the same pattern held for instrumental delivery and electronic fetal monitoring. A three-year study of midwife-attended home births in British Columbia also reported comparable perinatal death rates and severe neonatal complications in home and hospital births, as well as considerably fewer obstetric interventions in the home-birth group. Fewer severe perineal tears and hemorrhages occurred in the home-birth group (Janssen, Saxell et al., 2009).

Based on credible evidence indicating relative safety of home birth for mothers and newborns and lower rates of obstetric intervention (and associated risks), both the American College of Nurse Midwives (2005) and the American Public Health Association (2001) have issued policy statements supporting midwife-attended, planned home births. In contrast, in 2011, ACOG published a committee opinion opposing home births in response to findings indicating increased risk of neonatal death drawn largely from meta-analytic studies, the most recent of which (Wax, Pinette, & Cartin, 2010), if accurate, translated into a risk of about one extra neonatal death per 900 births (Tuffnell, 2010). Yet the otherwise strongly worded ACOG position statement that sparked a media storm opened on a decidedly more tentative note: "High quality evidence to inform the debate is limited" (ACOG, 2011b, p. 425).

It is in response to the limited "high quality evidence" informing professional opinions like ACOG's (2011b) that Keirse (2010), a professor of obstetrics, wrote, "Any new home birth study … is guaranteed to fuel the fires of controversy … shedding more heat than light on the subject" (p. 341). Keirse's comment arose partly from his identification of Wax and colleagues' (Wax et al., 2010) commission of serious research errors, which included selective exclusion of certain large-scale home-birth studies, mathematical errors, and reliance on birth certificate data that did not specify whether home birth was planned. In response to ongoing controversy and to the limitations of currently available scientific research on out-of-hospital birth, the British Health Service launched the Birthplace in England research initiative (National Perinatal Epidemiology Unit, 2011), a long-anticipated nationwide longitudinal study of home, center, and hospital birth outcomes and maternal perceptions.

By appearance, the controversy over professionally attended, planned home birth has as much to do with the relative values placed on maternal and fetal interests as on current evidence, particularly in light of research limitations. For example, the abstract and summary accompanying ACOG's (2011b) opinion recommend that mothers be fully informed of home birth's risks and benefits with specific reference to an increased risk of neonatal death. However, neither the abstract nor summary refers to research reviewed in the body of the paper that indicates increased rates of obstetric intervention in hospital birth with known consequences including, for example, twice the rate of cesarean delivery with its attendant increased risk of maternal mortality (see chapters 6 and 7), and the higher rate of perineal trauma in hospital birth than in home birth.

It has been argued that randomly assigning women to controlled home-birth versus hospital-birth treatments would definitively answer questions on outcomes associated with each, but few women would agree to be assigned (rather than choose) to give birth in a particular setting. In the one study involving random assignment, only 11 women participated (Dowswell, Thornton, Hewison, & Lilford, 1996), and the only noteworthy finding was hospital-birthing mothers' disappointment at having been assigned to hospital birth (Olsen & Jewell, 2009). In fact, any study involving randomly assigning mothers to one birth setting or another would apply only to the participants, as most women feel strongly about choosing where to deliver. Furthermore, even if more definitive data were to emerge showing increased neonatal mortality risk in home births, the difficult and fundamentally moral and ethical question of how to weigh one risk against another will remain.

In the meantime, it should be made plain that home birth offers mothers who choose to join a medical minority important nonmedical benefits, as indicated in studies conducted within and outside the United States. Across these studies, remarkable consistency in women's expressed rationale for choosing home birth arises; this reasoning includes maternal trust in childbirth as a natural and uncomplicated process, a desire to avoid unnecessary interventions, and the wish to give birth in a familiar environment. A study conducted in the Netherlands, where the home-birth rate is about 30% and thus represents a more culturally normative choice, corroborated the finding that home-birthing mothers wish to give birth in a familiar place (Borquez & Wiegers, 2006). Sjoblom, Nordstrom, and Edberg (2006) named the maternal desire to deliver in a familiar setting without unwanted interventions and women's faith in their bodies to safely give birth as components of "preserved maternal authority and autonomy" offered in out-of-hospital birth.

Women across the United States who chose planned home birth reported, like their international counterparts, that they preferred the home-birth approach because they wished to avoid unnecessary hospital obstetric procedures, adding their perception that many such procedures were unsafe, in turn making home birth safer than hospital delivery. In addition, U.S. respondents reported having chosen home birth in the wake of previous negative hospital experiences (Boucher, Bennett, McFarlin, & Freeze, 2009). One older U.S. study directly comparing planned home-birthing and hospital-birthing mothers found that indeed, more hospital-birthing mothers reported aversive experiences arising from intrusive medical procedures and the busy hospital environment (Hodnett, 1989).

STUDY MOTHERS ANTICIPATING PLANNED HOME OR CENTER BIRTH

Of the 75 mothers in this study, five (7%) were planning out-of-hospital births; four of the five were planning home births, and one mother was planning to deliver in a freestanding water-birth center. Two mothers were giving birth for the first time, and three were having their second babies. All mothers in this group had completed high school and two had college degrees. One mother was nonwhite. Income ranged from slightly above poverty to middle income; two mothers worked part time outside the home and one worked full time. One mother was uninsured, one had public health insurance, one had applied for public health insurance, and two had private insurance. All mothers were married or had stable partners. All mothers had contracted with certified midwives; one mother specified her attendant as a certified nurse-midwife, and another said her midwife was a naturopathic physician. Following the approach outlined in chapter 1, I discuss findings for the whole group, citing representative quotations and examples of experiences drawn directly from cases. Each case had a unique trajectory; therefore excerpts from each account are presented. Mothers' names are fictional.

In discussing their decisions to pursue out-of-hospital birth, mothers mentioned factors identified in previous studies, including desire for greater control in the birth process, wanting to give birth in a calm and peaceful environment, and trusting in the birth process as generally safe and uncomplicated. With one exception, all mothers mentioned without prompting feeling positively connected to and trusting their midwives; this sentiment is captured in second-time mother Melinda's statement, "I knew her personally before. I grew up with her daughters … [The midwives are] very calm, very trustworthy, very experienced."

Four of the five (80%) mothers reported having had family models of out-of-hospital birth as the primary guiding force in their decisions. In two cases, study mothers said they had witnessed their own mothers giving birth at home. For example, recalling several of her own mother's home births attended only by her father, Ellen said, "It was a good experience for me." Second-time mother Ginger had also witnessed several of her mother's home births attended by her father, and Ginger had been present for her sister's midwife-attended home birth, experiences that she said led her to choose the same childbirth pathway for herself. First-time mother Rosa, age 38, said her sister-in-law "came from Holland" and had given birth "calmly" at home in the United States.

Three experienced mothers based their out-of-hospital birth decisions partly on previous birth experiences; two of those had already had one home birth. Ginger described her first 12-hour, uncomplicated, home birth as "really short" and easy; in contrast, Melinda described her first home birth as "not easy … difficult, long" but remained committed to the approach. Second-time mother Carla described her out-of-hospital birth decision as largely a reaction to a negative first hospital-birth experience:

> Just because I was plus-sized … she [the obstetrician] … categorized me as high-risk … even though blood pressures were fine … Sure enough, as soon we get to the hospital I wasn't progressing fast enough for them … They said, "epidural or a c-section." Epidural came … they put me on oxygen … hooked [me] up to all kinds of machines. They were threatening c-section every time they turned around … That birth experience led me to become empowered.

Rosa, age 38, was the only mother to explicitly mention choosing out-of-hospital birth in the interest of avoiding cesarean delivery, saying, "I'm 38, almost 39. They just write you off as c-section, and I'll just die if I have that."

EXPECTATIONS OF MOTHERS PLANNING OUT-OF-HOSPITAL BIRTH

In describing expectations of childbirth, no mother directly mentioned an expectation of vaginal delivery, though such an expectation is implicit in this approach. Similarly, mothers did not directly address widely used obstetric procedures available only in hospitals, such as labor induction and acceleration with medications, pain medication (epidural or systemic), or the less frequently used instrument-aided birth. All mothers expected manual fetal monitoring, referring to "the Doppler," or stethoscope. Though all mothers said they fully expected to give birth in their selected setting attended by the midwives with whom they had originally contracted, Rosa was the only mother to allude to the possibility of emergency hospital care, saying, "My midwife is connected to a good hospital and good doctors. But I don't think it will come to that."

One expectation distinguishing this group from all others was the expectation of paying 50% or more of childbirth-related expenses. Ellen, who had no health insurance, said, "We're just paying … we really wanted to be able to pay for it on our own." Ginger had applied for public health insurance, but she said it was "tricky" to get coverage for home birth; still, she did not consider paying the full cost out of pocket "much of a worry." Melinda, who had private insurance, said she paid with cash because her insurance covered neither her midwife nor an out-of-hospital birth.

Among less frequently mentioned expectations were three mothers' explicit statements related to expecting childbirth pain, captured in Ellen's words, "I know it can be very painful. I know it's not going to be comfortable." The three experienced mothers did not expect amniotomy, whereas the two first-time mothers said they were unsure whether to expect it, but said they would willingly accept it upon their midwives' recommendations. Two experienced mothers said they expected natural tears, and Rosa, a first-time mother, said she had discussed episiotomy with her midwife and expected that the procedure "could" become part of her experience.

Other expectations were mentioned by only one mother each. First-time mother Ellen expected her experience to parallel what she had seen in her own mother's home births, saying, "There will be a point where I think I won't be able to make it ... After a little bit ... I'll want to start to push ... I'll lie down, or walk around ... squatting ... I like the idea of lying in bed." Having given birth once before, Melinda reported knowing "a little bit more" about what to expect with her upcoming birth. Only second-time mother Ginger expressly stated an expectation of a shorter labor this time around, saying she had noticed that in her own mother. Second-time mother Carla said she expected her upcoming birth to allow her "more freedom" and the comfort of birthing in water. No mothers mentioned expectations of serious childbirth or newborn complications.

Greatest Fears in Childbirth

Three (60%) mothers in this group cited newborn health as their chief childbirth-related worry, exemplified in Ginger's words, "I guess the same as every mom, [I worry] that everything goes okay. The baby comes out healthy with no problems, and they're breathing." Ellen raised a similar concern, saying she trusted her midwife to intervene appropriately, but newborn health was "still a worry."

Three (60%) mothers cited childbirth pain among their greatest childbirth worries; one mother had not previously given birth and the other two had. Melinda said, "Everybody goes through the pain. Since I know what's coming this time, I'm a little more worried." Further distinguishing these mothers from mothers expecting hospital vaginal birth was the absence of hospital-birthing mothers' oft-cited fear of possible cesarean delivery.

Summary of Out-of-Hospital Birthing Mothers' Expectations and Fears

All five mothers in this group expected to deliver in their chosen out-of-hospital setting attended by the midwives with whom they had contracted, with the expectation of vaginal delivery implicit but never directly stated. All five mothers expected manual fetal monitoring, but, consistent with their selected birth approach, mothers had no expectation of widely used hospital obstetric procedures such as medications to induce or accelerate labor or to treat labor pain. One hundred percent of mothers in this group expected to pay half or more of their total childbirth expenses, regardless of their insurance status. Less frequently, mothers mentioned expecting pain, episiotomy, experiences parallel to what they had witnessed, shorter labor than in a previous birth, and a more positive birth experience than a previous one. No mother in this group reported expecting serious maternal or newborn complications. Among mothers' fears were those common among hospital-birthing mothers, including worries about childbirth pain and newborn health.

Confirmed and Violated Expectations in Mothers Birthing Out of Hospital

Four (80%) of this chapter's five mothers gave birth outside hospitals as they had anticipated, but one of those four gave birth in her mother's rather than her own home as she had originally planned, leaving three of five (60%) mothers whose expectations of a specific birth setting were confirmed. Another mother experienced multiple expectancy violations—first, transport to the hospital and subsequently, multiple interventions, including IV opiates, epidural pain treatment, vacuum assistance, and episiotomy. All five (100%) mothers delivered vaginally.

Cases of Confirmed Expectations in Mothers Birthing Out of Hospital

All mothers who had expectations generally confirmed also experienced unanticipated events, which for second-time mother Melinda, involved an easier than anticipated birth with an unanticipated postpartum occurrence. During pregnancy, Melinda had said knowing what to expect worried her somewhat because her previous labor had been long, difficult, and painful. However, Melinda was pleasantly surprised to find her second birth experience shorter and less difficult than she had anticipated, leading her to say that things overall went "a lot better" than she had expected. She was not aware that she was in labor until a few hours before her newborn's arrival; Melinda contacted her midwives, who arrived shortly thereafter and helped her find comfort through walking, drinking juice, and finding a comfortable birth position "right away." Despite an unanticipated postpartum hemorrhage, Melinda reported feeling "grateful" for what she perceived as a "really easy birth," expressing confidence in her midwives' handling of her hemorrhage: "I could tell that they had experience with that before, so I wasn't nervous or scared … even that problem wasn't an issue."

By her description, first-time mother Ellen's birth proceeded much as her own mothers' home births had, though Ellen reported experiencing greater than expected childbirth pain. In labor 13 hours, Ellen said she "kept thinking" her labor was "a lot harder" than what she had witnessed, primarily because she "couldn't stand to talk" because of labor pain, for which she felt completely unprepared:

> I hadn't actually ever had anyone tell me it would hurt. And it hurt. And for the first couple days after I was like, "I'm not having any more children." I didn't think I did too good at it, but my mom and my midwife said I did very good for my first baby.

Surprising as she found her labor pain, Ellen said she "really appreciated" birthing in her own bed and in a generally quiet and comfortable environment. Overall, Ellen said, "It went very well and the way I wanted it to."

Carla, who had chosen a water-birth center in reaction to a previous negative hospital birth, described this birth as "perfect," despite being diagnosed in late pregnancy with pubic symphysis, a separation of the pelvic bones that resulted in severe pain, restricted movement, Carla's independent decision to forgo traditional medical treatment for the condition, and planning alternative birth positions. Carla said she reported to the water-birth center about two hours after her total five-hour labor had started. Her midwife checked Carla's and her fetus's conditions, and Carla then "got into the birth tub," where she stayed for a few hours. She started feeling "pushy," and after three pushes, "she [the baby] was out … born in the water." Overall, Carla said, "it was really, really great. I couldn't have asked for anything better … And that's why I chose the route that I did." Carla said her pain condition resolved within a few days postpartum, though her newborn required emergency care and a "series of more testing" for gastrointestinal problems beginning at about two weeks of age. Despite those problems, Carla described her newborn as "a good, happy, calm baby."

Case of Violated Expectation of Birth in Own Home

Though Ginger had expected and hoped to have a shorter labor than the 12 hours of her first birth, the duration of her labor this time stood as a testament to the adage *Be careful what you wish for*. Overall, Ginger said, her birth experience was "not at all" as she had expected. She had awakened in the middle of the night feeling "kind of funny," so Ginger called her mother and asked to go to her house to avoid waking her other child in her small apartment. "I actually started bleeding," Ginger said, so she woke her partner and child. "We got in the car and my water broke … I was pushing by the time I hit the door [of my mother's house] … My mom delivered him on the bed, moments later." Ginger had called her midwife before leaving her home, and they arrived after her labor "to deliver the placenta." In the total 29 minutes from "the first contractions to the last one," Ginger said, "luckily, everything was OK. I was expecting a short labor … [but] it was unbelievable."

Case of Violated Expectations of Home Birth with Hospital Birth and Interventions

In contrast to Ginger's 29-minute labor, Rosa said she labored at home for about 33 hours before her midwife said her fetus was "turned in such a way" that instrumental assistance appeared necessary. Rosa agreed to hospital transport, saying she felt she "needed extra help." Once in the hospital, Rosa said she readily accepted recommended IV medications and an epidural. Shortly after that, the attending obstetrician arrived, and "it was what I needed. The hospital bed was shaped [so] I could push … at home, I couldn't … The doctor was like a coach, just motivating me hard to keep on … a man's voice, the strength … it worked." Rosa said her midwife witnessed the obstetrician performing "a really good" episiotomy and using vacuum assistance "hardly at all" to ease her fetus out. Overall, Rosa said, she had no regrets about having planned home birth, believing that her midwives ultimately helped her get the best available care. She said she also felt certain that had she labored much longer in the hospital, any medical professional would "have gone for c-section right away, just because of my age … I just needed more help."

Satisfaction

Without exception, all mothers in this group reported feeling satisfied to highly satisfied with their birth experiences. All except one mother attributed the quality of their experiences to their midwives. Carla, whose expectation of delivering in a water-birth facility was confirmed, put it most simply: "I am very satisfied … It literally was everything that I wanted, and I remained, for the most part, in control the whole time. [My midwife] really gave me the freedom." Melinda, whose home-birth expectations were similarly confirmed, reported feeling "very satisfied" with her birth experience, attributing her positive experiences to midwives whom she perceived as "calm, reassuring," and knowledgeable. Ellen also spoke highly of her overall experience and of being "very impressed and happy" with her midwife. She added, "The cost was very nice."

The two mothers who experienced violated childbirth expectations both reported being satisfied or better; Rosa said she felt "very satisfied," adding, "I got to labor at home as long as I could. The midwives got me to the right hospital, the right doctor … It worked out the way it was supposed to."

In response to her precipitous labor, Ginger was the only mother in this group to qualify her overall satisfaction:

> He was happy and he was safe, and I was healthy and OK, so it was OK … I've definitely talked about being worried about having another child now … I'm just not planning on having another child any time in the near future … I know people usually don't ask to have longer labors … I was pretty scared when we were driving to my mom's house and my water broke, … thinking, "I'm going to deliver this baby in the car."

Summary and Implications

Fewer than 1% of 21st-century U.S. mothers consciously plan childbirth outside traditional hospitals, and according to national data, members of this maternal medical minority tend to be white and tend to be older, better educated, and better resourced than their average hospital-birthing counterparts. Though a general profile of relative advantage may apply to the overall population of U.S. mothers planning out-of-hospital birth, the five women in this study were diverse in terms of income and age, but all had at least a high school education. In contrast to their demographic diversity, one feature distinguished these mothers from others in this text: Regardless of their income or insurance status, these five stated ready willingness to cover half or more of the total costs of childbirth, and all expressed awareness that they would be paying more for out-of-home birth compared to hospital birth.

Another unifying distinction of this out-of-hospital birth group that has so far gone unreported in scholarly publications was that most mothers expressed having directly witnessed or learned about out-of-hospital birth from their own family members and that, in turn, those models positively influenced them in choosing the same path. This book's hospital-birthing mothers frequently referred to family members and friends influencing their childbirth decisions, but as often as not, hospital-birthing mothers chose a different path from that to which they had been exposed. Further evidence for the strength of mothers' immediate culture as a determining factor in the childbirth pathways they chose and anticipated lies in the fact that only one of this book's 70 hospital-birthing mothers spoke of any direct or indirect encounter with a mother who had planned out-of-hospital birth.

Beyond the unique influences on out-of-hospital birthing mothers' chosen childbirth pathway, their expectations otherwise paralleled those mentioned by hospital-birthing mothers expecting vaginal birth. Like hospital-birthing mothers, some out-of-hospital mothers expected pain, some expected shorter labors than previous ones (and had that expectation confirmed, even to an extreme), and others expected a better birth experience than a previous one. As did their hospital-birthing counterparts, a proportion of out-of-hospital birthing mothers saw their expectations violated. However, in contrast to hospital-birthing mothers anticipating low- or no-intervention birth, considerably more mothers birthing out of hospital had their expectations confirmed, with 60% giving birth out of hospital as anticipated and 80% delivering without intervention as expressly anticipated or implied. These figures starkly contrast with expectancy-confirmation rates in hospital no- or low-intervention groups, which could include hospital natural childbirth, VBAC, and "wait and see" mothers, groups for which expectancy confirmation reached a maximum of 40%.

It is often argued (e.g., ACOG, 2011b; Wax et al., 2010) that those attending planned out-of-hospital births carefully screen their patients for potential risk, and if any risk is identified, those patients are added to the pool of low-risk and higher risk hospital-birthing mothers. Therefore, hospital birth involves higher risk mothers who present more birth complications that require more interventions, which in turn violate expectations of no- or low-intervention birth among women who might have held them. Though difficult to dispute, this argument may be incomplete without any mention of the power or influence of maternal and professional expectations regarding the childbirth process.

Specifically, 100% of this chapter's mothers had an implicit expectation of vaginal birth, and perhaps because out-of-hospital birth equates to the absence of a surgical birth option, no mother mentioned personal concern that cesarean delivery might happen for her, in contrast to the frequency with which mothers in hospital vaginal-birth groups expressed that concern. Correspondingly, 100% of the out-of-hospital group's mothers delivered vaginally, including two mothers whose pregnancy status placed them in the category of high cesarean delivery probability (cf. Ecker & Frigoletto, 2007). One of these two, a second-time mother who described herself as "plus sized," had received a preeclampsia diagnosis in her previous birth and had been repeatedly reminded that cesarean delivery could become necessary while laboring in the hospital with her firstborn. The other mother was 38 years old and reported a labor of 38 hours, far exceeding a 12- or 20-hour standard of "normal" labor, and far exceeding the labor duration reported by every one of this study's hospital-birthing mothers who had anticipated vaginal birth but eventually delivered by cesarean. These two mothers' experiences underscore the need to attend to the quality of maternal expectations for childbirth and their power to affect its ultimate outcome, particularly in relationship to what the obstetric culture expects of mothers. From a scientific perspective, the mechanisms by which both maternal and professional obstetric expectations may exert their respective influences warrant careful attention.

Moreover, quantitative data on mothers planning out-of-hospital birth showing them to be socially advantaged (e.g., MacDorman et al. 2010) may present a misleading image of mothers giving birth in large, comfortable, privately owned homes. Although this study involved only five out-of-hospital birthing mothers, three described living in small rented apartments, two reported income at or just above the poverty level, and three had either no insurance or public health insurance. As much as any of this group's mothers might have struggled financially, however, all reported expecting (and being willing) to pay for at least half of their childbirth expenses, distinguishing them from other mothers possibly more profoundly than hard and fast demographic indicators do. Along with their expectation of paying at least half of their childbirth costs came these mothers' expectations of having the same person provide obstetric care throughout pregnancy and birth. Based on their reports of satisfaction, which all but one directly associated with her obstetric caregiver, this group's mothers seemed to believe that they got what they paid for in terms of the quality of the care they received and, in Melinda's report of competent treatment of her postpartum hemorrhage, in terms of caregiver knowledge and skill.

Another important distinction between out-of-hospital birthing mothers that goes beyond statistical indicators of low risk and social advantage was the conspicuous absence of any reference to recommended obstetric actions or to possibly having to accept particular unanticipated procedures for their own or their offspring's well-being. The absence of such reference became apparent in, for example, Carla's report of medical action surrounding her pubic symphysis, with her personal agency reflected directly in her statement, "My midwife and my chiropractor were both on board [with] just letting me, you know, kind of dictate what I wanted to do." Similarly, Rosa's story of accepting hospital transport after hours of laboring at home reflected her overall sense of agency in the decision and in subsequent steps.

Overall, these five out-of-hospital birthing mothers' accounts suggest that the potential negative impact of expectancy violations and unanticipated events can be buffered by factors beyond luck-of-the-draw physical performance in childbirth. First and foremost, all these mothers apparently and sufficiently trusted in the safety of the decision to join a tiny and controversial (at least in the United States, where hospital birth exists as an option) maternal medical minority. This unique characteristic should not be expected of all mothers, but it may in some way empower those in need of empowerment. Determination to have a birth experience of a certain quality, as in Carla's expressed desire for a better-than-previous birth and Rosa's determination to avoid cesarean delivery, seemed to play a role in at least those two mothers' birth processes and outcomes. Although no mother directly mentioned it, they all evidenced commitment to the out-of-hospital continuous care model offered by the midwives whose services they willingly paid for despite their financial circumstances; Melinda seemed to believe that this investment was fully justified by the competent treatment she received for postpartum hemorrhage.

As a long-term scientific goal, establishing the mechanisms by which factors—such as maternal views on the acceptability of out-of-hospital birth, maternal determination to achieve a desired experience, and maternal commitment to a specific model of care—may buffer unanticipated negative birth events certainly seems warranted. In the short term, an important lesson can be drawn from even this small number of maternal reports of satisfaction and the related perception of supportive and competent care. With the exception of Ginger's 29-minute labor, which no obstetric treatment could have prevented and which caused her lingering worries about future births, the remaining out-of-hospital mothers attached little ambivalence or equivocation to their childbirth experiences. First-time mother Ellen's statement is representative:

> I learned so much, I really wish other women would know … I'd tell them how nice birth can be … So many people … don't even think it's possible, don't even consider it; they think it's really weird … It was really nice to have a baby at home … They [women] can relax through it, get through [childbirth] without messing with their bodies, basically.

Chapter 9

Expectations and Experiences across Childbirth Pathways

The focus of this text is what women becoming mothers in the early 21st-century United States expected of labor and delivery, how their expectations matched their lived experiences, and how satisfied they were with the process overall. These questions seemed particularly pertinent in the complex and sometimes confusing context of contemporary maternal care, characterized by advancing obstetric technology, controversial views on the application of such technology, and the powerful influence of a health-care system under increasing strain. Using a qualitative approach mixing phenomenological and case study methods to examine the childbirth expectations and experiences of 75 women in individual interviews, I initially categorized accounts by the first thematic category to emerge, the particular childbirth pathway the mother reported anticipating. I then further analyzed maternal accounts within each pathway category, identifying childbirth expectations common to the entire subgroup and those unique to only a few mothers or to just one mother. The analytic approach permitted a matching of the expressed expectations to mothers' subsequent reported childbirth experiences at the level of the group and at the level of individual cases. The analytic approach also allowed a broader comparison between the respective subgroups, leading to implications drawn from the match between maternal expectations and the context in which mothers anticipated giving birth.

MORE ON IDENTIFYING EXPECTED CHILDBIRTH PATHWAYS

Mothers participating in this study were not intentionally recruited to represent any particular birth approach; rather, they had all responded to clinic and electronic advertisements for pregnant women interested in interviewing on their pregnancy and birth experiences. Recruitment sites were, however, selected with the intention of including demographically diverse women in order to more closely represent the contemporary population of birthing mothers. Reflecting that diversity, mothers' ages ranged from 19 to 43 years, and their education ranged from 8th grade to postgraduate; incomes ranged from poverty level to affluent, about 20–30% of each subgroup's mothers had public health insurance, and 21% of the overall sample was nonwhite. Most mothers were married or had stable partners.

Ascertaining how many contemporary women anticipate particular birth approaches or pathways on a national level for comparison purposes proved difficult because obstetric data are generally obtained from birth certificates; thus birth approaches are identified after the fact, rather than before. On those after-the-fact national obstetric indicators, my study sample mirrored the national profile (with a few exceptions). For example, among this study's 54 mothers expecting hospital vaginal delivery, 21 (39%) had labor induced, a figure remarkably similar to the 41% rate reported in 21st-century large-scale studies involving maternal reports (e.g., Declercq, Sakala, Corry, & Appelbaum, 2006). Also among the 59 mothers anticipating vaginal delivery, 29 (49%) reported receiving an epidural, within the 47–62% range reported across 19 U.S. states in 2006 (Osterman, 2009). Instrumental delivery was reported by one (1%) of the 59 mothers anticipating vaginal birth, again, consistent with national estimates (Martin et al., 2010). At 33%, the proportion of this study's mothers delivering by cesarean paralleled the early 21st-century reported 32% national rate (Martin et al., 2010). The five (7%) study mothers planning out-of-hospital birth considerably exceeded the national rate of about 1% (MacDorman, Menacker, & Declercq, 2010), likely reflecting both the relatively higher rate of out-of-hospital births in the two states from which the majority of interviewees came and out-of-hospital birthing mothers' interest in childbirth issues.

After-the-fact statistics on obstetric and birth outcomes such as labor induction, epidural administration, and cesarean delivery reflect the general state of maternal experiences and related care in a given place and time, and study data confirmed an overall high rate of technological intervention in birth. What such statistics cannot capture, however, is the process by which these procedures ultimately become part of women's individual childbirth stories, the explication of which stands to provide greater insight into women's individual experiences and into the state and evolution of the childbirth culture at large. In-depth studies like this one help fill a knowledge gap by revealing the dynamic nature of maternal expectations for specific childbirth pathways and related birth care and some of the processes involved in confirming expectations or sending them astray.

Deciding on Expected Childbirth Pathways

An initial factor involved in mothers' later childbirth experiences that reflected both their individual thinking and the larger obstetric culture was the decision on a childbirth pathway or approach. In particular, mothers described having settled on a birth approach as a function of their own values, their immediate cultural context (family and friends), and professional obstetric input, with the relative influence of each varying by approach and, for some, changing over time. For example, mothers seeking hospital natural childbirth described how their own values, family, and friends had influenced their childbirth plans, but only two mentioned any role of obstetric professionals in describing how previous supportive caregiving had influenced them to repeat the approach. In contrast, all mothers planning cesarean delivery, contemporary high-tech birth culture's flagship procedure, described obstetric professionals as playing a prominent role in their childbirth decisions. Most often, professional influence took the form of information provided on a medical risk involved in labor, such as possible breech position, placental problems, or rupture of a surgical scar. In some cases, the professional influence confirmed mothers' expressed preference for planned cesarean birth; in others, it conflicted with maternal desire for vaginal birth, VBAC, or mothers' families' objections to nonemergency surgery. Furthermore, some mothers switched from VBAC to planned cesarean based almost entirely on professional input. In all cases, professional input favoring planned cesarean ultimately became the deciding factor.

Whether influenced by family, friends, or medical professionals (or indirectly by insurance companies), few maternal decisions seemed completely autonomous, according to Dworkin's (1988) definition of autonomy as making decisions on one's own behalf for one's own reasons and motives rather than by the influence of external forces. Instead, across birth approaches, with some exceptions, mothers spoke of having arrived at their expected pathways in terms that suggested the women were falling into line with cultural expectations of them. For example, mothers describing their expectation of natural childbirth either in or outside of hospitals frequently referred to following a childbirth pathway that had been directly or indirectly modeled for them. For mothers planning out-of-hospital birth, the direct influence of family models in their decisions was most evident in the four of five mothers' reports of having witnessed or had contact with a family member who had delivered at home. First-time mothers planning an epidural spoke of family and friends who had encouraged them to plan the procedure based on their own positive experiences. The professional culture's apparent growing expectation of planned cesarean delivery when labor presents clear—or more often, potential—risks became evident in some maternal reports of having accepted the procedure despite personal misgivings.

Several mothers pursuing natural hospital childbirth and most of those pursuing VBAC stood out as having arrived at their expected childbirth pathway perhaps most autonomously. In the hospital-natural-childbirth group, multiple first- and later-time mothers reported long-standing, intuitive beliefs in intervention-free vaginal delivery as natural and healthy. All but one mother in the VBAC group expressed a similar belief, and those same four mothers had to translate those beliefs into actions, seeking available VBAC providers and signing papers indicating acceptance of VBAC risks.

Expecting mothers to plan childbirth pathways with complete autonomy and free of external influence would be unfair—for human beings are social creatures embedded in a sea of social influence—and would ignore the fact that they are making decisions with their fetuses in mind, about which little definitive can be known until their arrival as newborns. Under those circumstances, mothers are especially sensitive to both immediate and more distant social influences on their childbirth plans—as demonstrated, for example, in one mother's deciding on hospital rather than home birth in response to her husband's concern about something going awry, or in another's deciding to plan home birth in reaction to her familiarity with high rates of cesarean birth, a procedure she viewed as unsafe. More important, it is worth noting that by their accounts, mothers arrived at their decisions on and expectations for specific childbirth pathways with apparent thoughtfulness, rationality, and consideration for their own and others' needs. In some instances, maternal decisions may have, at least to some, appeared to compromise medical safety, as in Debra's (chapter 6) decision to forgo a scheduled cesarean so she could travel to another state to obtain help with her young children. One has to wonder whether knowledge that Debra made her decision based on the needs (including financial) of her whole family would have prompted Debra's obstetrician to treat her, as she might say it, with more respect.

MATERNAL EXPECTATIONS IN CONTEMPORARY CHILDBIRTH CULTURE

Chapter 2's figure 1 depicts graphically three pathways—hospital vaginal birth, out-of-hospital birth, and planned cesarean—drawn from maternal descriptions of childbirth expectations. Those pathways and their respective variations—for example, VBAC as a variation of hospital vaginal birth—aligned to a greater or lesser degree with the prevailing technocratic paradigm, characterized by an emphasis on technological intervention and physician-centered care and less emphasis on maternal participation and the quality of the mother–caregiver relationship (Davis-Floyd, 2001, 2004). The planned cesarean and planned epidural (a variation of hospital vaginal birth) pathways aligned most closely with the prevailing technocratic model. With an expectation of participating in childbirth and related medical decision making but with the reassurance of high-tech back-up care, mothers planning hospital natural birth or VBAC or those planning to "wait and see" on epidural administration aligned less with a technocratic and more with a humanistic care model. Most distant from the technocratic birth paradigm was the out-of-hospital childbirth pathway, which aligned instead with holistic care.

Although expected childbirth pathways generally aligned with either a technocratic, humanistic, or holistic treatment paradigm, closer analysis of detailed maternal expectations indicated that on an individual basis, some mothers fully subscribed to their pathway's respective orientation and others did not. For example, Iris (chapter 3) emphasized the importance of early epidural administration and obstetric caregiver technical skill and deemphasized the importance of relating to her caregiver, views closely aligned with the technocratic paradigm. Aligned with a holistic paradigm, Melinda (chapter 7) spoke of her practically lifelong personal relationship with her midwife as critical to her decision on and expectations of planned home birth. Other mothers' expressed expectations reflected a mixing of care orientations—for instance, mothers anticipating planned cesarean birth, arguably the most technocratic approach, also expected (or desired) a humanistic treatment component in the form of a birth attendant with whom they had an established relationship.

As mentioned in chapter 2, obstetric care has, in response to its own troubled history and general cultural shifts towards less authoritarian power structure (e.g., Genz, 2006), reoriented itself toward a mother-centered approach over the past half century, at least in terms of granting patients expressed rights to participate in treatment decisions. The shift away from traditional authoritarian structure in obstetric care should result in more humanistic care like that described by Davis-Floyd (2001, 2004) and can be seen in the increased availability of medical and nonmedical obstetric pain-relief options, more home-like birth-care settings, and more openness toward doula presence. But just as mothers are embedded in and subject to social influences, so is the obstetric community. As contemporary culture continues embracing (and paying for) technological solutions to physical health needs and conditions, the obstetric community will follow suit; this phenomenon is evidenced, for example, in increasing use of advanced fetal imaging technology that carries questionable medical benefit and in controversial applications of medical labor induction and planned cesarean delivery. Furthermore, contemporary value placed on fetal rather than maternal well-being (e.g., Douglas & Michaels, 2005; Hays, 1998) increases the risk that mothers will be sidelined in the service of technologically based, sometimes questionable approaches designed to ensure fetal well-being, such as intrapartum antibiotic prophylaxis (IAP; chapter 1).

Matches between Maternal Expectations, Experiences, and Birth Setting

Chapter 2's figure 1 indicates that, from the maternal perspective, hospital vaginal birth involves relatively more decision points and thus more opportunities for violation of expectations about birth attendant, labor onset, pain-relief and fetal monitoring strategies, and other commonly practiced hospital obstetric procedures. Consistent with the hypothesis that hospital vaginal birth could involve more expectancy violations, three of the four hospital vaginal-birth groups (natural, "wait and see," and VBAC) had the lowest expectancy-confirmation rates among all childbirth subgroups (table 1). Along the same lines, childbirth pathways involving fewer decision points—that is, planned cesarean delivery and out-of-hospital birth—had the highest expectancy-confirmation rates, exceeding the others by 20% or more. (Because one mother gave birth in her mother's home rather than her own home as had been planned, the expectation of the planned setting was technically violated, reducing the 80% expectancy-confirmation rate to 60%.) The one apparently anomalous result with respect to the hypothesis that fewer decision points would result in fewer opportunities for expectancy violation was the 59% expectancy-confirmation rate among the hospital vaginal birth "planned epidural" subgroup, a figure nearly 20% higher than those for the other two hospital vaginal birth subgroups.

As seen in chapter 4's maternal statements, expectations among mothers in the planned epidural subgroup generally adhered to a technocratic birth paradigm; these mothers expressed greater openness to technological intervention, such as labor induction and labor acceleration, compared to those in other vaginal birth subgroups. Predominantly technocratic, this group's expectations, like those of mothers planning cesarean delivery, matched the operating technocratic paradigm of the traditional

TABLE 1. Childbirth pathways, birth-setting paradigms, and expectancy-confirmation rates.

Mother's expected pathway	Childbirth pathway orientation	Birth-setting paradigm	Percent confirmed expectations
Hospital natural	Humanistic	Technocratic	38
VBAC	Humanistic	Technocratic	40
Wait and see	Humanistic	Technocratic	40
Spinal analgesia	Technocratic	Technocratic	59
Planned cesarean	Technocratic	Technocratic	62
Out of hospital	Holistic	Holistic	60–80

hospital institution. The match between technocratic expectations and technocratic care in the planned epidural and cesarean groups corresponded to the highest expectancy-confirmation rates of all study mothers. Likewise, mothers' expectations of an out-of-hospital birth pathway matched the out-of-hospital birth environment's holistic operating paradigm, and those mothers' expectancy-confirmation rates were as high as or higher than those for mothers on a technocratic pathway. Mothers whose expected childbirth pathways involved more humanistic or mixed humanistic-technocratic components (natural childbirth, VBAC, and even "wait and see") and took place in a technocratic setting—a mismatch—had the lowest expectancy-confirmation rates.

Expected Birth Approach, Expectancy Violations, and Birth Setting

Irrespective of whether mothers' expected childbirth pathways matched those of their planned birth settings, expectancy violations occurred in a sizeable percentage. Given the complexity of childbirth's physical process, many would find it unsurprising that mothers encounter some unexpected event over its course, a view voiced by multiple mothers who included among their reported childbirth expectations not knowing what to expect or expecting the unexpected. With their focus naturally on the childbirth process itself, most tend to associate "unexpected events" with a random physical occurrence, such as Ginger's surprise 29-minute labor (chapter 8), which no one could have likely predicted or controlled.

As much as violated expectations may symbolize randomness and unpredictability (e.g., Olson, Roese, & Zanna, 1996), patterns in the nature of expectancy violations emerged across and within childbirth subgroups. Among mothers whose expressed expectations aligned with the technocratic paradigm, violations related primarily to the limitations of technocratic care. For example, in the hospital birth with planned epidural group, nearly all expectancy violations involved the epidural procedure itself. In half the expectancy-violation cases, mothers did not receive the epidural as they had anticipated and were told either that their labor had progressed too far for analgesia administration (a curious claim, given that an epidural can technically be administered up until crowning) or that no anesthesiologist was available to perform the procedure. Among mothers who did receive spinal analgesia, several saw their expectations that it would ease the birth process violated by its lack of overall effectiveness or by highly aversive consequences requiring repeat hospitalization (see chapter 4). To ensure maximum efficiency in the delivery process, planned cesarean necessarily relies on tightly organized medical care, and violations mothers experienced of their expectations for planned cesarean delivery involved apparent organizational shortcomings as well as limitations of the procedures themselves. One planned cesarean mother experienced an unexpected excessive wait time, and two underwent labored cesareans not because their labors started before scheduled surgical dates or because of some other matter under their direct control but because their surgeries had never been scheduled owing to systemic issues.

In addition to direct expectancy violations resulting from shortcomings in technocratic care, mothers in the planned epidural and planned cesarean delivery groups experienced unanticipated events related to the care they did or did not receive. Not all such events were perceived negatively, at least in the immediate term, as in Ivey's (chapter 6) unexpected tummy tuck. However, most other unanticipated events reported in these two groups related to the technologically based procedures about which mothers had earlier expressed few concerns or in apparent problems within the care system. For example, Heather's (chapter 6) planned cesarean delivery proceeded much as she had expected, but she found herself distressed by her care system's lack of response to her repeated requests for breastfeeding assistance. Two mothers who planned an epidural (chapter 4) saw their previously expressed childbirth expectations generally confirmed but found themselves surprised by the variable course their highly managed labors took.

For mothers whose expected childbirth pathways aligned more with a humanistic approach, expectancy violations emerged primarily as consequences of the technocratic birth culture's routine responses to physical aspects of the birth process. As recounted by mothers planning hospital natural childbirth, the majority of those violations involved an obstetric caregiver's raising concern about an impending or recently passed due date for which the caregiver recommended labor induction as the solution. In most but not all cases, labor induction led to epidural administration, and in a few of those cases, cesarean delivery resulted. Mothers who experienced multiple expectancy violations, such as labor induction and epidural administration, shared the common feature of laboring in the hospital for more than 12 hours, excluding any time they may have labored outside hospital. In the "wait and see" group, a majority of expectancy violations (4 in 6) also began with labor induction, two cases of which led to labored cesarean. In the VBAC group, all expectancy violations involved cesarean delivery, planned in two cases and labored in a third.

By their descriptions, all mothers anticipating a humanistic childbirth pathway within a technocratic system were alerted by an obstetric professional of some medical concern that eventually led to the violations they experienced. Some medical concerns sounded less worrisome than others; compare, for example, news of "low amniotic fluid" as the reason for medical labor induction recommended within days of one's due date to the seemingly more urgent news of an elevated fetal heart rate as the reason for cesarean surgery. In nearly all cases, the news mothers received related to risk rather than to the certainty of some adverse outcome, and evidencing the guesswork involved in identifying some obstetric concerns are two mothers who accepted epidural analgesia upon their caregivers' warnings that they might be delivering babies larger than 10 pounds and who both had newborns weighing 7.5 pounds or less. However, at least by their reports, mothers did not generally question recommended maternal interventions at the time they received them but instead went along with their caregivers' recommendations.

When describing their childbirth experiences several months after the fact, however, some mothers questioned aspects of their birth care, focusing either on specific procedures or on larger institutional protocols.

For example, in the hospital-natural-childbirth group, Heidi (chapter 3) described distress that her obstetric caregiver had been preoccupied with adjusting an electronic fetal monitoring belt instead of checking on her labor progress—news of which Heidi believed would have helped her work through intense pain but the need for which she had difficulty communicating at the time. Also in chapter 3, Aisha, whose birth sounded to have proceeded as smoothly as one could imagine, questioned the necessity of the unanticipated 48-hour hospital stay that resulted in her transfer to an adult acute care ward because of overcrowding, protocol she did not question at the time. Crystal (chapter 4) stood out as one of the only mothers to take a firm stand against hospital protocol of slowing labor in order to ensure that an obstetrician would attend the delivery, but she also said both she and her husband had to do "a lot of convincing" to ensure that their wishes were respected.

One can easily see why, in the final days of pregnancy or under the stress of labor and with communication generally limited to discussion of medical risks and benefits (if even that), mothers comply with their caregivers' recommended courses of action. However, as the final receivers of such recommendations, mothers are left to make difficult decisions, such as whether to move forward with a recommended cesarean delivery. Unfortunately, as evidenced in some mothers' later questions about having followed medical recommendations or institutional protocol, doing so can cause lingering doubt or negativity toward the overall birth experience. Moreover, some mothers—for example, Alana (chapter 4), who responded to ineffective epidural analgesia with feelings of not having been assertive enough—take on more than their fair share of the responsibility for systemic or procedural shortcomings.

With little interference from larger institutions, the primary expectancy violations and unanticipated events faced by mothers on a holistic, out-of-hospital childbirth pathway involved physical occurrences in the birth process over which they or their caregivers had little direct control. Though unexpected physical events did occur, as in Melinda's postpartum hemorrhage and Rosa's protracted labor, for example, mothers reported little doubt or regret about their own decision making or about their midwives' handling of the situations. In comparison to hospital-birthing mothers, out-of-hospital birthing mothers made an apparent trade, maintaining less perceived control over childbirth's physical events but nearly complete control over the situational or practice aspects of obstetric care that caused expectancy violations and sometimes distress in their hospital-birthing counterparts.

Satisfaction

Most of this study's mothers reported being satisfied or better with their childbirth experiences. Not surprisingly, mothers whose expectations were confirmed reported feeling "very," "totally," or "completely" satisfied more often than mothers whose expectations were violated. Yet only a small proportion of mothers who saw expectations confirmed reported feeling satisfied without any further qualification, and with important exceptions, nearly all mothers who had expectations violated attached qualifications to their expressions of overall childbirth satisfaction.

This study's findings on qualified satisfaction as a function of expectancy violation are somewhat consistent with those of previous studies showing negative views of the birth experience corresponding to poorly matched expectations and experiences (Ayers & Pickering, 2005), including the introduction of unanticipated interventions (Slade, MacPherson, Hume, & Maresh, 1993). Along those lines, Penny (chapter 3) reported feeling "100% satisfied" but "with the exception" of having experienced labor induction, acceleration, and an epidural, none of which she had previously expected. Natalie (chapter 7) had originally planned VBAC and reported feeling "not that satisfied," attaching her feelings to having undergone a repeat cesarean and to apparent institutional disregard for aspects of her written birth plan.

Satisfaction statements also reflected mothers' relative orientations vis-à-vis technocratic, humanistic, or holistic birth care. For example, mothers expecting a largely technocratic, planned cesarean childbirth pathway generally referred to smooth and efficient institutional and surgical operation in describing overall satisfaction, whereas mothers who experienced institutional glitches referred directly to such glitches in qualifying their satisfaction statements. Reflecting a technocratic orientation in their planning for epidurals, mothers who did not receive analgesia as anticipated qualified their satisfaction statements, questioning whether their otherwise uncomplicated labors would have gone better with the procedure.

For mothers with a humanistic or holistic orientation, both of which acknowledge the person receiving medical care as central in making related decisions, the occurrence of previously unexpected procedures did not by itself necessarily correspond to lower or qualified satisfaction, but mothers' apparent involvement in deciding on such interventions did. For example, Shelly (chapter 3) described having undergone medical labor induction because her doctor "felt that it was important," and she qualified her satisfaction statement, saying she wished she had gone into labor naturally. In contrast, hospital-natural-childbirth mother Kayla (chapter 3), who experienced multiple expectancy violations including cesarean delivery, made reference only to a barely visible surgical scar when describing her overall satisfaction, perhaps because she herself requested surgery after a long, medically induced hospital labor. Similarly, Rosa (chapter 8), whose expectation of home birth was violated when she went to the hospital to obtain the "extra help" she felt she needed, attached no qualifications to satisfaction with her overall birth experience.

Taken in sum, this study's maternal reports reflect the importance of moving beyond a simple question of "how satisfied" one might have been with the complex experience of childbirth. Based on their responses only to the question of how satisfied they were overall, most (but not all) mothers reported being satisfied or better, but it has been suggested that instead of reflecting anything particularly positive, "satisfaction" may simply indicate one's view that nothing extremely bad happened (Williams, 1994). Along those lines, on the one hand, the satisfaction question did not by itself reveal the numerous instances mothers subsequently reported of supportive obstetric caregiving, an extreme example of which was Aisha's (chapter 3) report of her obstetrician's surprise return from vacation to attend her birth. On the other hand, the satisfaction question by itself did not capture equally important reported sources of distress for mothers who reported being otherwise satisfied. Those sources included unwanted but institutionally mandated hospital stays, mandated fetal monitoring procedures, poor staff response to requests for help, professional pressure to delay the urge to push the baby out, and inconsiderate staff behavior.

Redefining What to Expect

In the culture of preparing mothers and their caregivers for what to expect in childbirth, educational resources and programs generally focus on childbirth's physical aspects and medical and nonmedical ways of helping with normal or complicated birth (e.g., Armstrong, 2000; Murkoff & Mazel, 2008). As helpful as knowledge of labor and delivery events and related obstetric treatments may be, mothers could benefit from a broader consideration of what to expect in childbirth that addresses the types of situations associated with the expectancy violations encountered by many of this study's mothers. A more comprehensive view of what to expect seems particularly timely in a childbirth culture characterized by increasing emphasis on maternal responsibility for childbirth decisions and outcomes, an expanding menu of maternal childbirth options, and complex forces surrounding the obstetric care mothers receive.

In the context of rising obstetric intervention rates that show no signs of reversing, hospital-birthing mothers should in all fairness be prepared for the likelihood of receiving some unanticipated but relatively common obstetric intervention that either they had not previously considered or to which they had objected. Furthermore, mothers should be prepared to decide on recommended interventions based not on imminent threats to their own or their fetuses' well-being but on the risk that their status or condition may lead to a vaguely defined but undesired outcome. As an example, 21 (39%) mothers in this study had labor induced, the majority of whom stated during pregnancy that they neither anticipated nor felt positively about the procedure. In describing the medical rationale they received for labor induction, no study mother referred to any imminent threat to her own or her fetus's well-being; instead, mothers referred to vaguely defined risks, such as "low amniotic fluid" or an "old placenta," and only a handful reported what consequences their particular conditions might carry. In the absence of direct or imminent threat, perhaps it would be fairer for obstetric professionals who recommend procedures like labor induction or switching from planned VBAC to planned cesarean to then offer the mother several hours to consider the decision.

Though this may sound trite, it is worth reminding mothers of their hard-won right to refuse any recommended medical procedure, and it is worth encouraging mothers to say "No, thanks" to recommended procedures they oppose. However, this reminder comes with the understanding that advocating for oneself requires gathering the courage and presence of mind to do so, a difficult task under any circumstances and particularly challenging during the last few days of pregnancy or under the stress of labor. Some mothers in this study prepared themselves for potential professional or institutional challenges to their personal wishes by enlisting spouses, friends, or doulas to act as advocates or by preparing written birth plans. Even with such preparation, however, some mothers were asked to make quick decisions when, for example, obstetric caregivers recommended an epidural to help them relax during a long labor or recommended a cesarean to avoid "stressing the baby out." In the absence of better alternatives, perhaps it is best to simply prepare mothers for the prospect of on-the-spot, difficult decision making, reminding them that such situations are one of the unspoken costs of childbirth in the traditional technocratic and action-oriented hospital birth setting. Lastly, it is imperative to remind mothers that accepting an unanticipated medical recommendation in the disempowered state of being a hospital patient or a laboring person says more about the situation and constrained maternal choices than about a mother herself; criticism from oneself or from others about decisions made in childbirth is counterproductive to maternal well-being and healthy mother–child relations.

For mothers expecting childbirth involving advanced technology, expectations should address the likelihood that an anticipated technological intervention may fail to live up to its promise, as it did for mothers who received an epidural and found it ineffective (or only sporadically effective) and for mothers to whom the procedure was completely unavailable. Along similar lines, and in response to the absence of expressed concern among mothers regarding possible aversive consequences of upcoming technological procedures for themselves or their offspring, mothers anticipating technological intervention should be prepared for consequences such as those reported by study mothers, including possible dural puncture with an epidural or difficulties initiating breastfeeding following cesarean surgery. Although one perhaps naturally filters out details about possible undesirable consequences of any upcoming medical treatment, general and repeated reminders that technologically advanced procedures can go awry seem in order.

A longer term view on preparing mothers for what to expect in childbirth requires that the childbirth culture make some adjustments to its expectations of women. Though few could reasonably advocate a return to the day when medical practitioners made maternal medical decisions for women (supposedly in their best interests), the contemporary practice of alerting mothers to a sometimes ill-defined medical risk and then asking them to decide on a particular course of action does not seem to be the best or only alternative. As previously mentioned, providing time for a woman to consider the options may be appropriate in certain circumstances. Allowing a mother to immediately consult another obstetric caregiver may help in more pressing decisions, such as whether to pursue labored cesarean delivery. On a somewhat different note, given the occurrence of expectancy violations among mothers who labored in the hospital for more than 12 hours in the absence of serious childbirth complications (by their report), making hospital labor more tolerable seems to be in order. Drawing from reports of hospital-birthing mothers who spent most of their labors at home and from those of out-of-hospital birthing mothers, more tolerable labor would include the freedom to move, to drink as needed during labor, and to have a known caregiver present. As a more radical alternative, assigning a community nurse to check on laboring mothers in their homes until the final hours before delivery could prove safe, humane, and cost effective.

REVISITING RESEARCHER BIAS

In qualitative research, investigators are encouraged to actively reflect on their own views of the study topic partly to maximize prospects of fair data analysis (Moustakas, 1994; Sela-Smith, 2002). Throughout my numerous reads and analysis of maternal interview material, I kept in mind my existing view of contemporary birth culture as characterized by the same technological intrusion and chronic, anxiety-driven sense of time pressure present within 21st-century U.S. culture at large. As yet another example of the ever-increasing technological presence in childbirth, over the course of my writing this book, the U.S. cesarean rate crept up nearly a percentage point to just under 33%, another record high (Hamilton, Martin, & Ventura, 2010a, 2010b).

From an evolutionary perspective, human beings—human women and infants in particular—are robust. The species has survived over the millennia because its members can adapt to change, to perturbations in the contexts in which they operate. From that perspective, I found myself considering the expectation of a technocratic childbirth pathway as indicative of maternal adaptation to the prevailing technocratic childbirth paradigm, and that sort of adaptation carries several nonmedical benefits I had not previously considered. First, early acceptance of the technocratic model seemed to relieve some mothers of worries about childbirth pain or complications. For example, I could practically feel the relief expressed by mothers planning repeat cesarean partly based on their preference to avoid the negative labored cesarean experiences they had previously undergone. Another benefit of early acceptance of the technocratic paradigm appeared in a few mothers' reports of the confidence planned technological intervention gave them in achieving a good birth experience—Iris's declaration "Epidural, and I'm fine" quickly comes to mind. With some demonstrated association between positive expectations and positive outcomes (e.g., Christiaens, Verhaeghe, & Bracke, 2008;

Green, Coupland, and Kitzinger, 1990), a procedure's potential to boost maternal confidence should be included among its benefits in the overall risk calculation.

The multiple maternal reports of good experiences with technocratic birth led me to further consider the benefits of adapting to the prevailing technocratic model. I could not accept that mothers like Khala (chapter 3), who referred to childbirth with a planned epidural as "blissful," or like Ana (chapter 6), who described her planned cesarean delivery as "great," were somehow deluded or were fabricating their reports; I instead received their statements as rational expressions of positive impressions resulting from good birth experiences, or at least aspects of good birth experiences, involving advanced technology. As another related benefit of adapting to the prevailing technocratic birth paradigm, hospital-birthing mothers anticipating more technocratic birth pathways had higher rates of expectancy confirmation than other hospital-birthing mothers who expected less technocratic pathways.

On the other hand, from a systems perspective (e.g., Mitchell, 2009), adapting to a system that is being shaken up—shaken up in this case by introducing deviations into the natural childbirth process with technology—comes with consequences. Some of those consequences are immediate and obvious, such as Fae's (chapter 4) account of an "epidural nightmare" and Marta's (chapter 7) account of intense postsurgical pain. Some consequences are longer term, as in Carolyn's (chapter 6) description of placenta previa arising from a previous cesarean delivery and its worrisome complicating effects on her second pregnancy and birth. Other consequences are not immediately obvious but are nevertheless immediately registered by mothers, as evidenced in several reports of unanticipated and aversive experiences with internal fetal monitoring technology, including Michelle's (chapter 4) description of repeated attempts to place an electrode in her fetus's scalp.

Stating that expectation or acceptance of technocratic birth reflects adaptation to the childbirth culture at large implies that mothers who accept technocratic birth only partially or not at all were somehow less well adapted. In terms of raw numbers and percentages, the cost of mothers' lower level of adaptation to the technocratic birth environment (i.e., hospital) showed up in these women's higher rates of expectancy violation compared to mothers who expected a technocratic birth pathway early on. However, among mothers who expected a less technocratic birth pathway, the number and quality of unequivocally positive childbirth accounts rivaled that of the two technocratic childbirth subgroups, seen in, for example, Aisha's (chapter 3) report of an "amazing" birth experience and Annette's (chapter 7) report of feeling "ecstatic" over hers. Perhaps the prospect of such positive outcomes leads women like those featured in chapters 3, 6, and 7 to consciously decide against fully adapting to the prevailing technocratic birth paradigm and instead to carve a path more to their liking. The primary cost of taking these roads less traveled appears to be the risk of undergoing unanticipated technological intervention. Framing this risk as a consequence of following a path less aligned with the childbirth culture itself—and one that over the long term might help push that culture in a different direction—could help buffer against the distress or regret some hospital-birthing mothers expressed about having received unanticipated and undesired intervention.

Mothers apparently least adapted to the prevailing technocratic paradigm took the most dramatic turn away from that culture by planning childbirth to occur outside the traditional system. My own experience and this study's maternal reports have made me acutely aware that planning to participate in the out-of-hospital birth maternal medical minority requires the convergence of numerous forces. One's health in pregnancy, motivation, resources, and geographic location are but a few determining factors, and based on this study's maternal reports, direct contact with other out-of-hospital birthing mothers likely plays an important role, as well. The almost cosmic coming together of those forces does not occur for many mothers, and along with stating my frustration at that reality, I should also say that participating in a maternal medical minority is not for everyone. Nevertheless, it should be noted that out-of-hospital birthing mothers had the highest rate of expectancy confirmation and a closer read of their childbirth experiences indicated that on a case-by-case basis, these mothers spoke of their childbirth experiences in overwhelmingly positive terms. Maternal accounts also came as important reminders that home-birth attendants' formal training and hospital connections are critical components of a safe out-of-hospital birth experience.

As much as this study's maternal reports forced me to consider my own views on contemporary birth culture and women's roles within it, I found myself returning to a personal bias that trumps all others: Whichever childbirth pathway women follow, they deserve humane and respectful treatment. At times, I found myself angered by mothers' reports of having been pressured to accept what sounded like questionable—or worse, frankly inconsiderate—treatment, such as that described by Suzanne (chapter 4) or Debra (chapter 6). Such reports reinforced my view that hospital care can sometimes make the childbirth experience worse rather than better, and the risk of the former is particularly high when the institutions delivering obstetric services also have a financial stake in those services. At other times, I found myself applauding the kind, sometimes exceptional caregiving acts such as those described by Aisha and Courtney (chapter 3). Because mothers are ultimately the ones most directly affected by their childbirth experiences and will carry memories of them for the rest of their lives, this bias toward providing humane and respectful treatment must determine the future of maternal care.

Appendix

Comprehensive Expectant Mother Interview

Time 1: Third trimester of pregnancy

Mother's first name____________________:
Date of interview:_____________________:
Place of interview:____________________:

Introduction: Today's expectant mothers have more options than ever before. Even though today's advances are very exciting, keeping up with it all can be a lot. My goal is to hear your thoughts on your women's health-care experiences. To get a fuller picture of the moms in this study, I will also ask about your background.

Background

First question: What's your due date?
How was your due date calculated? (LMP, ultrasound?)
How many children have you previously had?
How is your pregnancy going so far?
What's the most exciting part about having this baby?
(If mother does not reveal: Was this pregnancy a surprise?)

Tell me a bit about the area you live in: Would you describe it as urban, suburban, or rural?

About how many people are in your community?

Are you living in an apartment, rental home, or a home you own?

Describe your family as it is today—who lives in your home and how you're related.

Tell me a little bit about how you grew up—maybe start with where you're from.
Who was in your family when you were growing up?
Who took care of you most of the time?
What kind of work did your parent(s) do?

General health

How would you describe your general health?
Before becoming pregnant, did you have any serious health problems?
PROBE questions:
At about what age did you have this problem?
How long did it last?
How did you learn you had this problem?
Tell me a little about your experiences with medical treatment for this problem.

Since becoming pregnant, have you had any serious health problems?
PROBE questions:
How did you learn you had this problem?
Tell me a little about your treatment for this problem.
How concerned are you now about this problem?
How are you dealing with this problem now?

Care questions

Would you say you get your prenatal care in a general family health clinic, a women's health clinic, or some other type of clinic?
If another type of clinic, please describe.

Is a doctor, midwife, or someone different in charge of your prenatal care?
How did you choose that person?
Do you usually see the same person at each visit? How are you with that situation?

About how visits many have you had?
About how much time did you spend with the doctor/midwife/other in each visit?
Would you say that was more time than you wanted to spend, about enough, or not enough time?
About how much time did you spend waiting for each visit?
About how much time did you spend getting to and from the visit?

(If applicable) Where are your other kids during your prenatal care appointments?

PROBE: How are you with that situation? (Etc.)

(If applicable) How easy is it for you to schedule prenatal care appointments around your home life?

(If applicable) Do you have to take time off work to go to the visit?

About how much time did you need to take off?
How do you work out your time off with your supervisor?
How easy or difficult is it for you to schedule prenatal care visits around your work?

Have you had ultrasound?
Have you had screening tests for birth defects (e.g., triple marker, amnio)?

If your pregnancy went a week or so past your due date, would you want to have your labor induced? Explain why.
How important is it for you to have the same person do your prenatal care and attend your delivery?
How important is having a vaginal delivery to you?
What kinds of things do you expect to happen when you go into labor?
What kinds of things do you expect to happen when you give birth?
What kinds of things do you not expect to happen when you go into labor?

What kinds of things do you not expect to happen when you give birth?
What do you most look forward to in childbirth?
What is your greatest worry about giving birth?
In what ways has your prenatal care prepared you (greatest fear, such as childbirth pain, etc.)?

Now I'm going to ask you to tell me whether you expect to have the following in labor and delivery.
A doctor or midwife you already know help you deliver your baby
Walk or move around during labor
Have ice chips during labor
Find a comfortable position during labor
Episiotomy
IV pain medication
Epidural pain treatment
Medications to speed up labor by making contractions quicker and more intense
Someone listen to baby's heartbeat from the outside with a stethoscope
Someone listen to baby's heartbeat from the outside using a monitoring machine
Someone insert a monitor into the birth canal to check baby's status
Induce labor with medications
Have your water broken
IV fluids during labor and delivery
Vaginal birth
Cesarean birth
Medical devices to help the baby through the birth canal
Hold the baby immediately after birth, before being weighed and checked over
Family members at the birth
Immunize the baby shortly after birth
Circumcise a male baby

Now to some questions about mental health and life situations that may have been part of your prenatal care:

Have you been asked about your mental health, such as stress or depression?

Have you been asked about family relations, including domestic violence?

Has seeing a therapist or counselor been part of your pregnancy care?

Finances

How do you pay for your prenatal care? (medical insurance, state medical plan, out of pocket)

How much of a worry is the actual cost of prenatal care for you?

Now, to our final questions. If you don't want to answer a question, say, "Skip it." (Skip any questions the mother has answered earlier in the interview.)

Your age (in years):	
Baby's father's age (in years):	
Do you have other children living in your home now?	◦ Yes ◦ No (skip to next question) Please list the sex, ages, and how you're related to each: (repeat as necessary for each child)
Do you currently work?	◦ Yes, full time. Your job is: ◦ Yes, part time. Your job is: ◦ No
What is your race or ethnicity?	◦ African American ◦ Asian American ◦ Hispanic or Latina ◦ Native American ◦ Mixed (specify): ◦ White or Caucasian ◦ Other (specify):

(*continued on next page*)

(*continued*)

Baby's father's race or ethnicity?	◦ African American ◦ Asian American ◦ Hispanic or Latino/a ◦ Native American ◦ Mixed (specify): ◦ White or Caucasian ◦ Other (specify):
How many years did you attend school?	◦ I went past 8th grade, but did not graduate ◦ I graduated from high school ◦ I went to college, but did not graduate ◦ I went to college for two years and graduated ◦ I went to college for four years and graduated ◦ I have a master's degree ◦ I have an advanced degree, such as MD, PhD, or JD
How many years did baby's father attend school?	◦ He went past 8th grade, but did not graduate ◦ He graduated from high school ◦ He went to college, but did not graduate ◦ He went to college for two years and graduated ◦ He went to college for four years and graduated ◦ He has a master's degree ◦ He has an advanced degree, such as MD, PhD, or JD
What is your approximate family income (all sources, per year)? *Read this list.*	◦ $0–25,000 ◦ $25,001–35,000 ◦ $35,001–50,000 ◦ $50,000–75,000 ◦ $75,001 and up
Who currently lives in your home (where you spend most of your time)? *Read list and check if mother says "yes."*	◦ Myself ◦ My other children ◦ My spouse/partner ◦ Other adults who are your blood relatives ◦ Other adults who are not blood relatives
Baby's father's job/ occupation:	
What is your relationship status?	◦ Married to baby's father. For how long? ◦ Cohabiting with baby's father. For how long? ◦ Not living with baby's father, but have contact ◦ Have no contact with baby's father

Comprehensive Maternal Interview

Time 2: Two months postpartum

Mother's first name____________________:
Date of interview:_____________________:
Place of interview:____________________:

Introduction: Now that your baby is here, I'm going to ask you questions about how you're doing and about your birth experience. Any questions before we start?

When was your baby born?
What was your baby's birth weight?
How close was your baby's actual birth date to your due date?
The last time I spoke with you was about before your due date. In those weeks, did anything significant happen in your health or medical care?
Has anything changed in the following since we last talked?

Change in spouse or partner
new people living in your house (besides newborn)
significant change in your income
significant change in your job
significant change in your baby's father's job
major changes in your health

General health

How would you describe your general health today?
How would you describe your baby's general health today?
Has your baby's health improved, stayed about the same, or gotten worse since birth?

Now some questions about your labor and delivery.

Where did you give birth to your baby?
About how long were you in labor?

Tell me how things went once you knew you were in labor.
Who was with you during your labor?
And during the actual delivery?
How was your birth experience similar to your expectations?
How was your birth experience different from your expectations?
Did you have any birth complications? Please explain.
How long were you in the hospital?
Since your baby was born, have you…
Been given education on breastfeeding?
Been asked about your emotional state, such as your stress level or depression?

ASK ONLY IF MOM HAD C-SECTION:
Describe how the decision was made for you to have a c-section.
How much control do you feel like you had in the decision?

Interactions with Medical Providers

Which type of medical provider helped you deliver your baby?
How well did you know that person before delivering your baby?
How comfortable were you asking your (doctor, nurse, midwife) questions during your labor?
How well did your (doctor, nurse, midwife) answer your questions?
How much were you able to make decisions during your baby's birth?
Did your (doctor, nurse, midwife) recommend anything you didn't agree with?
In general, how satisfied are you with your labor and delivery experience? If you could go back and make anything go differently, what might that be?

Now I'm going to ask you to tell me whether you had any of the following things during labor and delivery. (Ask only as needed.)

Had someone you already know help deliver your baby
Walked or moved around during labor
Had ice chips during labor
Found a comfortable position during labor
Had episiotomy
Had IV pain medication
Had epidural pain treatment
Had medications to speed up labor
Someone listened to baby's heartbeat with a stethoscope
Attached a belt around the abdomen to get fetal heartbeat
Inserted a monitor into the birth canal to check baby's status
Induced labor with medications
Had water broken
Had IV fluids during labor and delivery
Vaginal birth
Cesarean birth
Medical devices were used to help the baby through the birth canal
Held the baby immediately after birth, before baby was weighed and checked over
Family members attended the birth
Immunized the baby shortly after birth
Circumcised a male baby

Feeding

How did you feed your baby today (past 24 hours)? (PROMPTS: breastfeed exclusively, used pumped milk, formula, bottles)

Finances

How satisfied are you with the financial part of your labor and delivery?
How did you pay for your pregnancy care? (private insurance, medical coupons, out of pocket)

Looking back

Now that you're a few months past your birth experience, is there anything you learned that you think might be helpful to share with other mothers-to-be?

And are there things you learned during your prenatal care that you think would be helpful to share with other mothers-to-be?

References

Alfirevic, Z., Devane, D., & Gyte, G. M. (2006). Continuous cardiotocography (CTG) as a form of electronic fetal monitoring (EFM) for fetal assessment during labour. *Cochrane Database of Systematic Reviews*, Issue 3, Art. No.: CD006066. doi:10.1002/14651858.CD006066.

Alfirevic, Z., Kelly, A. J., & Dowswell, T. (2009). Intravenous oxytocin alone for cervical ripening and induction of labour. Cochrane *Database of Systematic Reviews*, Issue 4, Art. No.: CD003246. doi:10.1002/14651858.CD003246.pub2.

Ali, U. A., & Norwitz, E. R. (2009). Vacuum-assisted vaginal delivery. *Reviews in Obstetrics and Gynecology, 2*(1), 5–17.

American College of Nurse Midwives. (2005). Position statement on home birth. Washington, DC: American College of Nurse Midwives. Retrieved from http://www.midwife.org/siteFiles/position/homeBirth.pdf.

American College of Nurse Midwives. (2009). Position statement: Nitrous oxide for labor analgesia. Silver Spring, MD: American College of Nurse Midwives. Retrieved from http://www.midwife.org/siteFiles/position/Nitrous_Oxide_12_09.pdf.

American College of Obstetricians and Gynecologists [ACOG]. (1999). ACOG practice bulletin (No. 5, July 1999, replaces practice bulletin No. 2, October 1998). Vaginal birth after previous cesarean delivery. Clinical management guidelines for obstetrician-gynecologists. *International Journal of Gynecology & Obstetrics, 66*(1), 197–204.

American College of Obstetricians and Gynecologists [ACOG]. (2008). *Code of professional ethics of the American College of Obstetricians and Gynecologists.* Washington, DC: ACOG.

American College of Obstetricians and Gynecologists [ACOG]. (2009). ACOG practice guideline (No. 107, August 2009): Induction of labor. *Obstetrics and Gynecology, 114*(2, Part 1), 386–397.

American College of Obstetricians and Gynecologists [ACOG]. (2010). ACOG practice bulletin (No. 115, August 2010, replaces practice bulletin No. 54, July 2004 and committee opinion Number 342, August 2006). Vaginal birth after previous cesarean delivery. Clinical management guidelines for obstetrician-gynecologists. *International Journal of Gynecology & Obstetrics, 116*(2, Part 1), 450–463.

American College of Obstetricians and Gynecologists [ACOG], Office of Communications. (2011a). OB-Gyns issue less restrictive VBAC guidelines. Retrieved from http://www.acog.org/from_home/publications/press_releases/nr07–21-ten-1.cfm.

American College of Obstetricians and Gynecologists [ACOG]. (2011b). Planned home birth. Committee Opinion No. 476. *Obstetrics and Gynecology, 117*(2, Part 1), 425–428.

American College of Obstetricians and Gynecologists [ACOG] & American Society of Anesthesiologists [ASA]. (2004). Pain relief during labor. ACOG Committee Opinion No. 295. American College of Obstetricians and Gynecologists. *Obstetrics & Gynecology, 104*(1), 213.

American Medical Association. (1990). Fundamental elements of the patient-physician relationship. *Journal of the American Medical Association, 264*(24), 3133–3134.

American Public Health Association. (2001). Increasing access to out-of hospital maternity care services through state-regulated and nationally-certified direct-entry midwives (APHA Policy Statement #20013). Retrieved from http://mana.org/APHAformatted.pdf.

American Society of Anesthesiologists Task Force on Obstetric Anesthesia [ASATFOA]. (2007). Practice guidelines for obstetric anesthesia. *Anesthesiology*, *106*(4), 843–863.

Anderson, R. E., & Anderson, D. A. (1999). The cost-effectiveness of home birth. *Journal of Nurse Midwifery, 44*(1), 30–35.

Anim-Somuah, M., Smyth, R., & Howell, C. (2005). Epidural versus nonepidural or no analgesia in labour. *Cochrane Database of Systematic Reviews*, Issue 4, Article No.: CD000331. doi:10.1002/14651858.CD000331.pub2.

Anonymous. (1977). The pregnant patient's bill of rights. *MCN: The American Journal of Maternal Child Nursing, 2*(2), 137–138.

Arms, S. (1975). *Immaculate deception: A new look at women and childbirth in America.* Boston: Houghton Mifflin.

Armstrong, E. (2000). Lessons in control: Prenatal education in the hospital. *Social Problems, 47*(4), 583–605.

Ayers, S., & Pickering, A. D. (2005). Women's expectations and experience of birth. *Psychology and Health, 20*(1), 79–92.

Bahl, R., Patel, R. R., Swingler, R., Ellis, M., & Murphy, D. J. (2007). Neurodevelopmental outcome at 5 years after operative delivery in the second stage of labor: A cohort study. *American Journal of Obstetrics & Gynecology, 197*(2), 147.e1–147.e6.

Baltimore, R. S. (2007). Consequences of prophylaxis for group B streptococcal infections of the neonate. *Seminars in Perinatology, 31*(1), 33–38.

Benzon, H., Raja, S. N., Molloy, R. E., Liu, S., & Fishman, S. M. (2004). *Essentials of pain medicine and spinal labor analgesia* (2nd ed.). New York: Churchill Livingston/Elsevier.

Berghella, V., Baxter, J. K., & Chauhan, S. P. (2008). Evidence-based labor and delivery management. *American Journal of Obstetrics & Gynecology, 199*(5), 445–454.

Berghella, V., Blackwell, S. C., Ramin, S. M., Sibai, B. M., & Saade, G. R. (2011). Use and misuse of the term "elective" in obstetrics. *Obstetrics & Gynecology, 117*(2, Part 1), 372–376.

Betrán, A. P., Merialdi, M., Lauer, J. A., Bing-shun, W., Thomas, J., Van Look P. et al. (2007). Rates of caesarean section: Analysis of global, regional and national estimates. *Paediatric Perinatology and Epidemiology, 21*(2), 98–113.

Block, J. (2008). *Pushed: The painful truth about childbirth and modern maternity care.* Cambridge, MA: Da Capo Press.

Booth, C. and Meltzoff, A. (1984). Expected and actual experience in labour and delivery and their relationship to maternal attachment. *Journal of Reproductive and Infant Psychology, 2*(2), 79–91.

Borquez, H., & Wiegers, T. (2006). A comparison of labour and birth experiences of women delivering in a birthing centre and at home in the Netherlands. *Midwifery, 22*(4), 339–347.

Boucher, D., Bennett, C., McFarlin, B., & Freeze, R. (2009). Staying home to give birth: Why women in the United States choose home birth. *Journal of Midwifery and Women's Health, 54*(1), 119–126.

Boylan, P. C. (1989). Active management of labor: Results in Dublin, Houston, London, New Brunswick, Singapore, and Valparaiso. *Birth, 16*(3), 114–118.

Brown, H. C., Paranjothy, S., Dowswell, T., & Thomas, J. (2008). Package of care for active management in labour for reducing caesarean section rates in low-risk women. *Cochrane Database of Systematic Reviews,* Issue 4, Art. No.: CD004907. doi:10.1002/14651858.CD004907.pub2.

Campbell, O. M., & Graham, W. J. (2006). Strategies for reducing maternal mortality: Getting on with what works. *The Lancet Online.* doi:10.1016/S0140-6736(06)69381-1.

Carlton, T., Callister, L. C., & Stoneman, E. (2005). Decision making in laboring women: Ethical issues for perinatal nurses. *Journal of Perinatal and Neonatal Nursing, 19*(2), 145–154.

Carroli, G., & Mignini, L. (2009). Episiotomy for vaginal birth. *Cochrane Database of Systematic Reviews*, Issue 1. Art. No.: CD000081. doi:10.1002/14651858.CD000081.pub2.

Carter, F. A., Frampton, C. M., & Mulder, R. T. (2006). Cesarean section and postpartum depression: Examining the link. *Psychosomatic Medicine, 68*(2), 321–330.

Caton D. (2009). The history of obstetric anesthesia. In: D. H. Chestnut, L. S. Polley, L. C. Tsen, & C. A. Wong (Eds.), *Obstetric Anesthesia Principles and Practice* (4th ed.) (pp. 3–13). Philadelphia: Elsevier Mosby.

Caughey, A. B., Sandberg, P. L., Zlatnik, M. G., Thiet, M. P., Parer, J. T., & Laros, R. K. (2005). Forceps compared with vacuum: Rates of neonatal and maternal morbidity. *Obstetrics and Gynecology, 106*(5, Part 1), 908–912.

Caughey, A. B., Sundaram, V., Kaimal, A. J., Cheng, Y. W., Gienger, A., Kaimal A. J. et al. (2009, March). *Maternal and neonatal outcomes of elective induction of labor*. Evidence Report/Technology Assessment No. 176. (Prepared by the Stanford University-UCSF Evidenced-based Practice Center under contract No. 290–02–0017.) AHRQ Publication No. 09-E005. Rockville, MD: Agency for Healthcare Research and Quality.

Chang, K. Y., Chan, K. H., Chang, S. H., Yang, M. C., & Chen, T. H. (2008). Decision analysis for epidural labor analgesia with multiattribute utility (MAU) model. *Clinical Journal of Pain, 24*(3), 265–272.

Chourasia, V. S., & Tiwari, A. K. (2008). A review and comparative analysis of recent advances in fetal monitoring techniques. *Critical Reviews in Biomedical Engineering, 36*(5–6), 335–373.

Christiaens, W., Verhaeghe, M., & Bracke, P. (2008). Childbirth expectations and experiences in Belgian and Dutch models of maternity care. *Journal of Reproductive and Infant Psychology, 26*(4), 309–322.

Cicchetti, D., Rogosch, F. A., & Toth, S. L. (1998). Maternal depressive disorder and contextual risk: Contributions to the development of attachment insecurity and behavior problems in toddlerhood. *Development and Psychopathology, 10*(2), 283–300.

Clark, S. L., Belfort., M. A., Byrum, S. L., Myers, J. A., & Perlin, J. B. (2008). Improved outcomes, fewer cesarean deliveries, and reduced litigation: Results of a new paradigm in patient safety. *American Journal of Obstetrics & Gynecology, 199*(2), 105e.1–105e.7.

Clark, S. L., Belfort, M. A., Dildy, G., A., Herbst, M. A., Meyers, J. A., & Hankins, J. D. (2008). Maternal death in the 21st century: Causes, prevention, and relationship to cesarean delivery. *American Journal of Obstetrics and Gynecology, 199*(1), 36.e1–36.e5.

Clark, S. L., Belfort., M. A., Dildy, G. A., & Myers, J. A. (2008). Reducing obstetric litigation through alterations in practice patterns. *Obstetrics and Gynecology, 112*(6), 1279–1283.

Clark, S. L., Simpson, K. R., Knox, G. E., & Garite, T. J. (2009). Oxytocin: New perspectives on an old drug. *American Journal of Obstetrics and Gynecology, 200*(1), 35.e1–35.e6.

Coco, A., Derksen-Schrock, A., Coco, K., Raff, T., Horst, M., & Hussar, E. (2010). A randomized trial of intravenous hydration in labor when oral fluid is unrestricted. *Family Medicine, 42*(1), 52–56.

Cohen J. (1996). Doctor James Young Simpson, Rabbi Abraham De Sola, and Genesis chapter 3, verse 16. *Obstetrics and Gynecology, 88*(5), 895–898.

Colb, S. F. (2004). Crying murder when a woman refuses a c-section: The disturbing implications of a Utah prosecution. Retrieved from http://writ.news.findlaw.com/colb/20040316.html.

Collis, R. E., Davies, D. W., & Aveling, W. (1995). Randomized comparison of combined spinal-epidural and standard epidural analgesia in labour. *Lancet, 345*(8962), 1413–1416.

Cone, T. E. (1979). *History of American pediatrics.* Boston: Little, Brown & Co.

Crowe, K. & von Baeyer, C. (1989). Predictors of a positive childbirth experience. *Birth, 16*(2), 59–63.

Cunningham, F. G., Bangdiwala, S., Brown, S. S., Dean, T. M., Frederiksen, M., Rowland-Hogue, C. J. et al. (2010, March 8–10). National Institutes of Health Consensus Development Conference Statement: Vaginal birth after cesarean: New insights. *Obstetrics and Gynecology, 115*(6), 1279–1295.

Cunningham, F., Leveno, K., Bloom, S., Hauth, J., Rouse, D., & Spong, C. (2009). *Williams obstetrics* (23rd ed.). New York: McGraw-Hill Professional.

Curtin, S. D., & Park, M. M. (1999). Trends in the attendant, place and timing of births, and in the use of obstetric interventions: United States, 1989–97. *National Vital Statistics Reports, 47*(27). Hyattsville, MD: National Center for Health Statistics.

Dannenbring, D., Stevens, M. J., & House, A. E. (1997). Predictors of childbirth pain and maternal satisfaction. *Journal of Behavioral Medicine, 20*(2), 127–142.

Daskalakis, G., Anastasakis, E., Papantoniou, N., Mesogitis, S., Thomakos, N., & Antsaklis, A. (2007). Cesarean vs. vaginal birth for term breech presentation in 2 different study periods. *International Journal of Gynecology & Obstetrics, 96*(3), 162–166.

Davis-Floyd, R. (2001). The technocratic, humanistic, and holistic paradigms of childbirth. *International Journal of Gynecology & Obstetrics, 75*(Supplement 1), S5–S23.

Davis-Floyd, R. (2004). *Birth as an American rite of passage* (2nd ed.). Berkeley: University of California Press.

Declercq, E., Barger, M., Cabral, H. J., Evans, S. R., Kotelchuk, M., Simon, C. et al. (2007). Maternal outcomes associated with planned primary cesarean births compared with planned vaginal births. *Obstetrics and Gynecology, 109*(3), 669–677.

Declercq, E., MacDorman, M. F., Menacker, F., & Stotland, N. (2010). Characteristics of planned and unplanned home births in 19 states. *Obstetrics and Gynecology, 116*(1), 93–99.

Declercq, E., Menacker, F., & MacDorman, M. F. (2006). Maternal risk profiles and the primary cesarean rate in the United States, 1991–2002. *American Journal of Public Health, 96*(5), 867–872.

Declercq, E. R., Sakala, C., & Corry, M. P. (2002). *Listening to mothers I: Results of the first national U.S. survey of women's childbearing experiences.* New York: Maternity Center Association/Harris Interactive.

Declercq, E. R., Sakala, C., Corry, M. P., & Appelbaum, S. (2006). *Listening to mothers II: Results of the second national U.S. survey of women's childbearing experiences.* New York: Childbirth Connection. Retrieved from http://www.childbirthconnection.org/listeningtomothers/.

Deering, S. H., Zaret, J., McGaha, K., & Satin, A. J. (2007). Patients presenting with birth plans: A case control study of delivery outcomes. *Journal of Reproductive Medicine, 52*(10), 884–887.

DeFrances, C. J., Cullen, K. A., & Kozak, L. J. (2007). National Hospital Discharge Survey: 2005 annual summary with detailed diagnosis and procedure data. *National Center for Health Statistics. Vital Health Statistics, 13*(165). Retrieved from http://www.cdc.gov/nchs/data/series/sr_13/sr13_165.pdf.

Donahue, E., Brooten, D., Roncoli, M., Arnold, L., Knapp, H., Borucki, L., & Cohen, A. (1994). Acute care visits and rehospitalization in women and infants after cesarean birth. *Journal of Perinatology, 14*(1), 36–40.

Douglas, S. J., & Michaels, M. W. (2005). *The mommy myth: The idealization of motherhood and how it has undermined all women.* Tampa, FL: Free Press.

Dowswell, T., Thornton, J.G., Hewison , J., & Lilford, R. J. (1996). Should there be a trial of home versus hospital delivery in the United Kingdom? Measuring outcomes other than safety is feasible. *British Medical Journal, 312*(7033), 753.

Dublin, S., Lyndon-Rochelle, M., Kaplan, R. C., Watts, D. H., & Critchlow, C. W. (2000). Maternal and neonatal outcomes after induction of labor without an identified indication. *American Journal of Obstetrics & Gynecology, 183*(4), 986–994.

Dudding, T. C., Vaizey, C. J., & Kamm, M. A. (2008). Obstetric anal sphincter injury: Incidence, risk factors, and management. *Annals of Surgery, 247*(2), 224–237.

Dworkin, G. (1988). *The theory and practice of autonomy.* New York: Cambridge University Press.

Ecker, J. L., & Frigoletto, F. D. (2007). Cesarean delivery and the risk-benefit calculus. *New England Journal of Medicine, 356*(9), 885–888.

Eisenach, J. C., Pan, P. H., Smiley, R., Lavand'homme, P., Landau, R., & Houle, T. T. (2008). Severity of acute pain after childbirth, but not type of delivery, predicts persistent pain and postpartum depression. *Pain, 140*(1), 87–94.

Epstein, R. H. (2010). *Get me out: A history of childbirth from the Garden of Eden to the sperm bank.* New York: Norton.

Fenwick, J., Gamble, J., & Hauck, Y. (2007). Believing in birth—Choosing VBAC: The childbirth expectations of a self-selected cohort of Australian women. *Journal of Clinical Nursing, 16*(8), 1561–1570.

Fiske, S. T., & Taylor, S. E. (1991). *Social cognition* (2nd ed.). New York: McGraw-Hill.

Foureur, M., Ryan, C. L., Nicholl, M., & Homer, C. (2010). Inconsistent evidence: Analysis of six national guidelines for vaginal birth after cesarean section. *Birth, 37*(1), 3–10.

Freedman, L. Z., & Ferguson, V. M. (1950). The question of "painless childbirth" in primitive cultures. *American Journal of Orthopsychiatry, 20*(2), 363–379.

Freedman, R. M., & Baltimore, R. (1990). Fatal streptococcus viridans septicemia and meningitis: Relationship to fetal scalp electrode monitoring. *Journal of Perinatology, 10*(3), 272–274.

Frigoletto, F. G., Lieberman, E., Lang, J., Cohen, A., Barrs, V., Ringer, S. et al. (1995). A clinical trial of active management of labor. *New England Journal of Medicine, 333*(12), 745–750.

Fuglenes, D., Oian, P., & Kristiansen, I. S. (2009). Obstetricians' choice of cesarean delivery in ambiguous cases: Is it influenced by risk attitude or fear of complaints and litigation? *American Journal of Obstetrics & Gynecology, 200*(1), 48.e1–48.e8.

Fulop-Miller, R. (1938). *Triumph over pain.* New York: Literary Guild of America.

Gamble J., & Creedy, D. (2000). Women's request for a cesarean section: A critique of the literature. *Birth, 27*(4), 256–263.

Gamble J., & Creedy, D. (2001). Women's preference for a cesarean section: Incidence and associated factors. *Birth, 28*(2), 101–110.

Gamble, J., Creedy, D. K., McCourt, C., Weaver, J., & Beake, S. (2007). A critique of the literature on women's request for cesarean section. *Birth, 34*(4), 331–340.

Geller, E. J., Wu, J. M., Jannelli, M. L., Nguyen, T. V., & Visco, A. G. (2010). Neonatal outcomes associated with planned vaginal versus planned primary cesarean delivery. *Journal of Perinatology, 30*(4), 258–264.

Genz, S. (2006). Third way/ve: The politics of postfeminism. *Feminist Theory, 7*(3), 333–353.

Gibbins, J., & Thomson, A. M. (2001). Women's expectations and experiences of childbirth. *Midwifery, 17*(4), 302–313.

Glaser, B. G. (1978). *Theoretical sensitivity: Advances in the methodology of grounded theory.* Mill Valley, CA: Sociology Press.

Goldberg, A. B., Cohen, A., & Lieberman, E. (1999). Nulliparas' preferences for epidural analgesia: Their effects on actual use in labor. *Birth, 26*(3), 139–143.

Gottvall, K., & Waldenstrom, U. (2002). Does a traumatic birth experience have an impact on future reproduction? *BJOG: An International Journal of Obstetrics & Gynaecology, 109*(3), 254–260.

Graham, H. (1951). *Eternal Eve: The history of gynaecology and obstetrics.* New York: Doubleday.

Granroth, G. (1979). Defects of the central nervous system in Finland. IV. Associations with diagnostic X-ray examinations. *American Journal of Obstetrics & Gynecology, 133*(2), 191–194.

Green, J. M., & Baston, H. H. (2003). Feeling in control in labor: Concepts, correlates and consequences. *Birth, 30*(4), 235–247.

Green, J. M., & Baston, H. A. (2007). Have women become more willing to accept obstetric interventions and does this relate to mode of birth? Data from a prospective study. *Birth, 34*(1), 6–13.

Green, J. M., Coupland, V. A., & Kitzinger, J. V. (1990). Expectations, experiences, and psychological outcomes of childbirth: A prospective study of 825 women. *Birth, 17*(1), 15–24.

Green, J. M., Coupland, V. A., & Kitzinger, J. V. (1998). *Great expectations: A prospective study of women's expectations and experiences of childbirth.* Cheshire, England: Books for Midwives.

Grivell, R. M., Alfirevic, Z., Gyte, G. M., & Devane, D. (2010). Antenatal cardiotocography for fetal assessment. *Cochrane Database of*

Systematic Reviews, Issue 1, Art. No.: CD007863. doi:10.1002/14651858.CD007863.pub2.

Guise, J.-M., Eden, K., Emeis, C., Denman, M. A., Marshall, N., Fu, R., Janik, R., Nygren, P., Walker, M., & McDonagh, M. (2010). Vaginal birth after cesarean: New insights. Evidence Report/Technology Assessment No. 191. (Prepared by the Oregon Health and Science University Evidence-based Practice Center under Contract No. 290–2007–10057-I). AHRQ Publication No. 10-E003. Rockville, MD: Agency for Healthcare Research and Quality. Retrieved from http://www.ahrq.gov/downloads/pub/evidence/pdf/vbacup/vbacup.pdf.

Hall, M. H., & Bewley, S. (1999). Maternal mortality and mode of delivery. *Lancet, 354*(9180), 776.

Hall, M. J., DeFrances, C. J., Williams, S. N., Golosinskiy, A., & Schwartzman, A. (2010). National Hospital Discharge Survey: 2007 summary. *National health statistics reports, 29*. Hyattsville, MD: National Center for Health Statistics. Retrieved from http://www.cdc.gov/nchs/data/nhsr/nhsr029.pdf.

Hamilton, B. E., Martin, J. A., & Ventura, S. J. (2010a, April). Births: Preliminary data for 2008. *National vital statistics reports web release, 58*(16). Retrieved from http://www.cdc.gov/nchs/data/nvsr/nvsr58/nvsr58_16.pdf.

Hamilton, B. E., Martin, J. A., & Ventura, S. J. (2010b). Births: Preliminary data for 2009 *National Vital Statistics Reports, 59*(3). Retrieved from http://www.cdc.gov/nchs/data/nvsr/nvsr59/nvsr59_03.pdf.

Hawkins, J. L., Gibbs, C. P., Orleans, M., Martin-Salvaj, G., & Beaty, B. (1997). Obstetric anesthesia workforce survey, 1981 versus 1992. *Anesthesiology, 87*(1), 135–143.

Hays, S. (1998). *The cultural contradictions of motherhood.* Cambridge, MA: Yale University Press.

Heinze, S. D., & Sleigh, M. J. (2003). Epidural or no epidural anaesthesia: Relationships between beliefs about childbirth and pain control choices. *Journal of Reproductive and Infant Psychology, 21*(4), 323–333.

Henderson, J., & Petrou, S. (2008). Economic implications of home births and birth centers: A structured review. *Birth, 35*(2), 136–146.

Hildingsson, R., Radestad, I., Rubertsson, C., & Waldenstrom, U. (2002). Few women wish to be delivered by caesarean section. *BJOG: An International Journal of Obstetrics & Gynaecology, 109*(6), 618–623.

Hinova, A., & Fernando, R. (2009). Systemic remifentanil for labor analgesia. *Anesthesia and Analgesia, 109*(6), 1925–1929.

Hodnett, E. D. (1989). Personal control and the birth environment: Comparisons between home and hospital settings. *Journal of Environmental Psychology, 9*(3), 207–216.

Holloway, I. (2008). *A–Z of qualitative research in healthcare* (2nd ed.). Oxford: Blackwell.

Hoyert, D. L. (2007). Maternal mortality and related concepts. *National Center for Health Statistics. Vital and Health Statistics 3*(33). Washington, DC: U.S. Department of Health and Human Services. Retrieved from http://www.cdc.gov/nchs/data/series/sr_03/sr03_033.pdf.

Impey, L. (1999). Maternal attitudes to amniotomy and labor duration: A survey in early pregnancy. *Birth, 26*(4), 211–214.

Jackson, N., & Paterson-Brown, S. (2001). Physical sequelae of cesarean section. *Best Practice and Research: Clinical Obstetrics & Gynaecology, 15*(1), 49–61.

Janssen, P. A., Henderson, A. D., & Vedam, S. (2009). The experience of planned home birth: Views of the first 500 women. *Birth, 36*(4), 297–304.

Janssen, P. A., Lee, S. K., Ryan, E. M., Etches, D. J., Farquharson, D. F., Peacock, D. et al. (2002). Outcomes of planned home births versus planned hospital births after regulation of midwifery in British Columbia. *Canadian Medical Association Journal, 166*(3), 315–323.

Janssen , P. A., Saxell, L., Page, L. A., Klein, M. C., Liston, R. M., & Lee, S. K. (2009). Outcomes of planned home birth with registered midwife versus planned hospital birth with midwife or physician. *Canadian Medical Association Journal, 181*(6–7), 377–383.

Johanson, R. B., Heycock, E., Carter, J., Sultan, A. H., Walklate, K., & Jones, P. W. (1999). Maternal and child health after assisted vaginal delivery: Five year follow up of a randomised controlled study comparing forceps and ventouse. *BJOG: An International Journal of Obstetrics & Gynaecology, 106*(6), 544–549.

Johnson, K. C., & Daviss, B. A. (2005). Outcomes of planned home births with certified professional midwives: Large prospective study in North America. *British Medical Journal, 330*(7505), 1416.

Kannan, S., Jamison, R. N., & Datta, S. (2001). Maternal satisfaction and pain control in women electing natural childbirth. *Regional Anesthesia and Pain Medicine, 26*(5), 468–472.

Kaufman, T. (2007). Evolution of the birth plan. *Journal of Perinatal Education, 16*(3), 47–52.

Keirse, M. J. (2010). Home birth: Gone away, gone astray, and here to stay. *Birth, 37*(4), 341–346.

Kieser, K. E., & Baskett, T. A. (2002). A ten year population based study of uterine rupture. *Obstetrics & Gynecology, 100*(4), 749–753.

Kukla, R. (2005). Conscientious autonomy: Displacing decisions in health care. *Hastings Center Reports, 35*(2), 34–44.

Kukla, R., Kuppermann, M., Little, M., Lyerly, A. D., Mitchell, L. M., Armstrong E. M. et al. (2009). Finding autonomy in birth. *Bioethics, 23*(1), 1–8.

Kuklina, E. V., Meikle, S. F., Jamieson, D. J., Whiteman, M. K., Barfield, W. D., Hillis, S. D., & Posner, S. F. (2009). Severe obstetric morbidity in the United States: 1998–2005. *Obstetrics & Gynecology, 113*(2, Part 1), 293–299.

Lamaze, F. (1970). *Painless childbirth: The Lamaze method.* Chicago: Henry Regnery.

Landau, R. (2009). Pain relief during labor. *F1000 Medicine Reports, 1*(5). doi:10.3410/M1-5.

Lang, C. T., & King, J. C. (2008). Maternal mortality in the United States. *Best Practice and Research: Clinical Obstetrics and Gynaecology, 22*(3), 517–531.

Lauer, J. A., Betrán, A. P., Merialdi, M., & Wojdyla, D. (2010). Determinants of cesarean section rates in developed countries: Supply, demand and opportunities for control. *World Health Report Background Paper No. 29.* Retrieved from http://www.who.int/healthsystems/topics/financing/healthreport/29DeterminantsC-section.pdf.

Lederman, R. P., Lederman, E., Work, B., & McCann, D. S. (1985). Anxiety and epinephrine in multiparous labor: Relationship to duration of labor and fetal heart rate pattern. *American Journal of Obstetrics & Gynecology, 153*(8), 870–877.

Lee, K. S. (2007). Infant mortality decline in the late 19th and early 20th centuries: The role of market milk. *Perspectives in Biology and Medicine, 50*(4), 585–602.

Lee, K. S., Paneth, N. Gartner, L. M., Pearlman, M. A., & Gruss, L. (1980). Neonatal mortality: An analysis of the recent improvement in the United States. *American Journal of Public Health, 70*(1), 15–21.

Leeman L., Fontaine, R, King, V., Klein, M. C., & Ratcliffe, S. (2003a). The nature and management of labor pain, part 1: Non-pharmacologic pain relief. *American Family Physician, 68*(6), 1109–1112.

Leeman L., Fontaine, R., King, V., Klein, M. C., & Ratcliffe, S. (2003b). The nature and management of labor pain, part 2: Pharmacologic pain relief. *American Family Physician, 68*(6), 1115–1120.

Lothian, J. A. (2001). Do birthing options really exist? *Journal of Perinatal Education, 10*(3), viii–xi.

Loudon I. (1987). Puerperal fever, the streptococcus, and the sulphonamides, 1911–1945. *British Medical Journal, 295*(6596), 485–490.

Loudon, I. (1992). *Death in childbirth: An international study of maternal care and maternal mortality, 1800–1950*. New York: Oxford University Press.

Luke, B., Williams, C., Minogue, J., & Keith, L. (1993). The changing pattern of infant mortality in the U.S.: The role of prenatal factors and their obstetrical implications. *International Journal of Gynecology & Obstetrics, 40*(3), 199–212.

Lurie, S. (2005). The changing motives of cesarean section: From the ancient world to the twenty-first century. *Archives of Gynecology and Obstetrics, 271*(4), 281–285.

Lurie, S., Feinstein, M., Hofetz, C., & Mamet, Y. (1999). Iatrogenic bacterial meningitis after spinal anesthesia for pain relief during labor. *Journal of Clinical Anesthesia, 11*(5), 438–439.

MacDorman, M. F., & Mathews, T. J. (2008). Recent trends in infant mortality in the United States. *National Center for Health Statistics Data Brief, No. 9*. Hyattsville, MD: National Center for Health Statistics. Retrieved from http://www.healthypeople.gov/document/HTML/Volume2/16MICH.htm#_Toc494699662.

MacDorman, M. F., Menacker, F., & Declercq, E. (2008). Cesarean birth in the United States: Epidemiology, trends, and outcomes. *Clinics in Perinatology, 35*(2), 293–307.

MacDorman, M. F., Menacker, F., & Declercq, E. (2010). Trends and characteristics of home and other out-of-hospital births in the United States, 1990–2006. *National Vital Statistics Reports, 58*(11). Hyattsville, MD: National Center for Health Statistics. Retrieved from http://www.cdc.gov/nchs/data/nvsr/nvsr58/nvsr58_11.PDF.

Martin, J. A., Hamilton, B. E., Sutton, P. D. (2009). Births: Final data for 2006. *National Vital Statistics Reports, 57*(7). Hyattsville, MD: National Center for Health Statistics. Retrieved from *www.cdc.gov/nchs/data/nvsr/nvsr57/nvsr57_07.pdf.*

Martin, J. A., Hamilton, B. E., Sutton, P. D., Ventura, S. J., Mathews, T. J., Kirmeyer, S. et al. (2010). Births: Final data for 2007. *National Vital Statistics Reports, 58*(24). Hyattsville, MD: National Center for Health Statistics. Retrieved from http://www.cdc.gov/nchs/data/nvsr/nvsr58/nvsr58_24.pdf.

Martin, J. A., Hamilton, B. E., Sutton, P. D., Ventura, S. J., Menacker, F., & Kirmeyer, S. (2006). Births: Final data for 2004. *National Vital Statistics Reports, 55*(1). Hyattsville, MD: National Center for Health Statistics. Retrieved from *www.cdc.gov/nchs/data/nvsr/nvsr55/nvsr55_01.pdf.*

McGrath, P., Phillips, E., & Vaughan, G. (2010). Speaking out! Qualitative insights on the experience of mothers who wanted a vaginal birth after a birth by cesarean section. *The Patient: Patient-Centered Outcomes Research, 3*(1), 25–32.

McMahon, M. J., Luther, E. R., Bowes, W. A., & Olshan, A. F. (1996). Comparison of a trial of labor with an elective second cesarean section. *New England Journal of Medicine, 335*(10), 689–695.

Meddings, F., Phipps, F. M., Haith-Cooper, M., Haigh, J. (2007). Vaginal birth after cesarean section (VBAC): Exploring women's perceptions. *Journal of Clinical Nursing, 16*(1), 160–167.

Meikle, S. F., Steiner, C. A., Zhang, J., & Lawrence, W. L. (2005). A national estimate of elective primary cesarean delivery rate. *Obstetrics and Gynecology, 105*(4), 751–756.

Melzack R. (1984). The myth of painless childbirth (The John J. Bonica lecture). *Pain, 19*(4), 321–337.

Melzack, R. (1993). Labour pain as a model of acute pain. *Pain, 53*(2), 117–120.

Menacker, F. (2005). Trends in cesarean rates for first births and repeat cesarean rates for low-risk women: United States, 1990–2003. *National Vital Statistics Reports, 54*(4). Hyattsville, MD: National Center for Health Statistics. Retrieved from *www.cdc.gov/nchs/data/nvsr/nvsr54/nvsr54_04.pdf.*

Menacker, F., Declercq, E., & MacDorman, M. F. (2006). Cesarean delivery: Background, trends and epidemiology. *Seminars in Perinatology, 30*(5), 235–241.

Menacker, F., & Hamilton, H. E. (2010). Recent trends in cesarean delivery in the United States. NCHS data brief, no 35. Hyattsville, MD: National Center for Health Statistics. Retrieved from *http://www.cdc.gov/nchs/data/databriefs/db35.pdf.*

Menacker, F., MacDorman, M. F., & Declercq, E. (2010). Neonatal mortality risk for repeat cesarean compared to vaginal birth after cesarean (VBAC) deliveries in the United States, 1998–2002 birth cohorts. *Maternal Child Health Journal, 14*(2), 147–154.

Menacker, F., & Martin, J. A. (2009). BirthStats: Rates of cesarean delivery, and unassisted and assisted vaginal delivery, United States, 1996, 2000, and 2006. *Birth, 36*(2), 167.

Miller, D. T., & Turnbull, W. (1986). Expectancies and interpersonal processes. *Annual Review of Psychology, 37*(1), 233–256.

Mitchell, M. (2009). *Complexity: A guided tour.* New York: Cambridge University Press.

Moleti, C. A. (2009). Trends and controversies in labor induction. *Maternal Child Nursing, 34*(1), 40–47.

Moustakas, C. (1994). *Phenomenological research methods.* Thousand Oaks, CA: Sage.

Mozurkewich, E., Chilimigras, J., Koepke, E., Keeton, K., & King, V. J. (2009). Indications for induction of labour: A best evidence review. *BJOG: An International Journal of Obstetrics & Gynaecology, 116*(5), 626–636.

Mozurkewich. E., & Wolf, F. M. (2000). Near-infrared spectroscopy for fetal assessment during labour. *Cochrane Database of Systematic Reviews*, Issue 3. Art. No.: CD002254. doi:10.1002/14651858. CD002254.

Mueller-Heubach, E. (2007). The pursuit of evidence. *American Journal of Obstetrics & Gynecology, 196*(4), 366–372.

Murkoff, H., & Mazel, S. (2008). *What to expect when you're expecting* (4th ed.). New York: Workman.

Murphy, D. J., & Koh, D. K. (2007). Cohort study of the decision to delivery interval and neonatal outcome for emergency operative vaginal delivery. *American Journal of Obstetrics & Gynecology, 196*(2), 145.e1–145.e7.

Murphy, D., J., Liebling, R. E., Verity, L., Swingler, R., & Patel, R. (2001). Early maternal and neonatal morbidity associated with operative delivery in second stage of labour: A cohort study. *Lancet, 358*(9289), 1203–1207.

Namey, E. E., & Lyerly, A. D. (2010). The meaning of "control" for childbearing women in the U.S. *Social Science & Medicine, 71*(4), 769–776.

National Perinatal Epidemiology Unit. (2011). Birthplace in England research programme. Retrieved from http://www.npeu.ox.ac.uk/birthplace.

Nguyen, U. D., Rothman, K. J., Demissie, S., Jackson, D. J., Lang, J. M., & Ecker, J. L. (2010). Epidural analgesia and risks of cesarean and operative vaginal deliveries in nulliparous and multiparous women. *Maternal Child Health Journal, 14*(5), 705–712.

Nystedt, A., Edvardsson, D., & Willman, A. (2004). Epidural analgesia for pain relief in labour and childbirth—A review with a systematic approach. *Journal of Clinical Nursing, 13*(4), 455–466.

O'Hara, M. W. (1987). Post-partum "blues," depression, and psychosis: A review. *Journal of Psychosomatic Obstetrics and Gynecology, 7*(3), 205–227.

Ohlsson, A., & Shah, V. S. (2009). Intrapartum antibiotics for known maternal group B streptococcal colonization. *Cochrane Database of Systematic Reviews*, Issue 3. Art. No.: CD007467. doi:10.1002/14651858.CD007467.pub2.

Olde, E., van der Hart, O., Kleber, R., & van Son, M. (2006). Post-traumatic stress following childbirth: A review. *Clinical Psychology Review, 26*(1), 1–16.

Olsen, O., & Jewell, D. (2009). Home versus hospital birth. *Cochrane Database of Systematic Reviews, 998*, Issue 3, Art. No.: CD000352. doi:10.1002/14651858.CD000352.

Olson, J. M., Roese, N. J., & Zanna, M. P. (1996). Expectancies. In E. T. Higgins & A. W. Kruglanski (Eds.), *Social psychology: Handbook of basic principles* (pp. 211–238). New York: Guilford.

Osterman, M. J. (2009). BirthStats: Percentage of mothers receiving epidural/spinal anesthesia by age, race, & Hispanic origin of mother: Total of 18 reporting areas, singletons only, 2006. *Birth, 36*(4), 340–341.

Osterman, M. J., Martin, J. A., & Menacker, F. (2009). Expanded health data from the new birth certificate, 2006. *National Vital Statistics Reports, 58*(5). Hyattsville, MD: National Center for Health Statistics. Retrieved from http://www.cdc.gov/nchs/data/nvsr/nvsr58/nvsr58_05.pdf.

O'Sullivan, G., & Scrutton, M. (2003). NPO during labor. Is there any scientific validation? *Anesthesiology Clinics of North America, 21*(1), 87–98.

Pace, M. C., Aurilio, C., Bulletti, C., Iannotti, M., Passavanti, M B., & Palagiano, A. (2004). A comparison of subarachnoid analgesia and pudendal block in advanced labor: Analgesic quality and obstetric outcome. *Annals of the New York Academy of Sciences, 1034*, 356–363.

Pang, P. W., Leung, T. N., Lan, T. K., & Hang Chung, T. K. (2008). Impact of first childbirth on changes in maternal preference for mode of delivery: Follow-up of a longitudinal observational study. *Birth, 35*(2), 121–128.

Pates, J. A., & Satin, S. J. (2005). Active management of labor. *Obstetrics and Gynecology Clinics of North America, 32*(2), 221–230.

Perl, L. M. (2010). The birth and death of VBACs in a rural community hospital. *Birth, 37*(3), 257–258.

Perlow, J. H., Wigton, T., Hart, J., Strassner, H. T., Nageotte, M. P., & Wolk, B. M. (1996). Birth trauma: A five-year review of incidence and associated perinatal factors. *Journal of Reproductive Medicine, 41*(10), 754–760.

Phillips, E., McGrath, P., & Vaughan, G. (2009–2010). 'I wanted desperately to have a natural birth': Mothers' insights on vaginal birth after cesarean (VBAC). *Contemporary Nurse, 34*(1), 77–84.

Pitcock, C. D. & Clark, R. B. (1992). From Fanny to Fernand: The development of consumerism in pain control during the birth process. *American Journal of Obstetrics & Gynecology, 167*(3), 581–587.

Poole, J. H. (2003). Neuraxial analgesia for labor and birth: Implications for mother and fetus. *Journal of Perinatal and Neonatal Nursing, 17*(4), 252–267.

Powell, J., Gilo, N., Foote, M., Gil, K., & Lavin, J. P. (2007). Vacuum and forceps training in residency: Experience and self-reported competency. *Journal of Perinatology, 27*(6), 343–336.

Ramsey, P. S., Ramin, K. D., & Ramin, S. M. (2000). Labor induction. *Current Opinion in Obstetrics and Gynecology, 12*(6), 463–473.

Rawal, N., van Zundert, A., Holmström, B., & Crowhurst, J. A. (1997). Combined spinal-epidural technique. *Spinal Labor Analgesia and Pain Medicine, 22*(5), 406–423.

Read, G. D. (1944). *Childbirth without fear.* New York: Harper & Brothers.

Reynolds, F. (2010). The effects of maternal labour analgesia on the fetus. *Best Practice and Research: Clinical Obstetrics and Gynaecology, 24*(3), 298–302.

Rich, A. (1976). *Of woman born: Motherhood as experience and institution.* New York: Norton.

Roberts, R. G., Deutchman, M., King, V. J. Fryer, G. E., & Miyoshi, T. J. (2007). Changing policies on vaginal birth after cesarean: Impact on access. *Birth, 34*(4), 316–323.

Roberts, S. P., & Petts, H. V. (1990). Meningitis after obstetric spinal anaesthesia. *Anaesthesia, 45*(5), 376 –377.

Robinson, J. & Godbey, G. (2005). Time in our hands. *The Futurist, 39*(5), 18–22.

Rooks, J. P. (2007). Nitrous oxide for pain in labor—Why not in the United States? *Birth, 34*(1), 3-5.

Rosen, M. A. (2002). Nitrous oxide for relief of labor pain: A systematic review. *American Journal of Obstetrics & Gynecology, 186*(5, Supplement), S110–S126.

Rozen, G., Ugoni, A. M., & Sheehan, P. M. (2011). A new perspective on VBAC: A retrospective cohort study. *Women and Birth: Journal of the Australian College of Midwives, 24*(1), 3–9.

Rubin, M. M. (2007). Antenatal exposure to DES: Lessons learned ... future concerns. *Obstetric & Gynecological Survey, 62*(8), 548–555.

Sakala, C. (2006). Carol Sakala's letter from North America: An uncontrolled experiment: Elective delivery predominates in the United States. *Birth, 33*(4), 332–335.

Sakala, C., & Corry, M. P. (2008). Evidence-based maternity care: What it is and what it can achieve. Retrieved from http://www.milbank.org/reports/0809MaternityCare/0809MaternityCare.html#sidebar4.

Sandelowski, M. (1995). Sample size in qualitative research. *Research in Nursing and Health, 18*(2), 179–183.

Shachar, I. B., & Weinstein, D. (1998). High risk pregnancy outcome by route of delivery. *Current Opinion in Obstetrics and Gynecology, 10*(6), 447–452.

Schultz, D. G. (Ed). (1958, May). Cruelty in maternity wards. *Ladies' Home Journal, 75,* 44–45, 152.

Segal, S. (2010). Labor epidural analgesia and maternal fever. *Anesthesia and Analgesia, 111*(6), 1467–1475.

Sela-Smith, S. (2002). Heuristic research: A review and critique of Moustakas's method. *Journal of Humanistic Research, 42*(3), 53–88.

Shorten, A. (2010). Bridging the gap between mothers and medicine: "New insights" from the NIH consensus conference on VBAC. *Birth, 37*(3), 181–183.

Simkin, P. (1992). Just another day in a woman's life? Part II: Nature and consistency of women's long-term memories of their first birth experiences. *Birth, 19*(2), 64–81.

Simkin, P., & Bolding, A. (2004). Update on nonpharmacologic approaches to relieve labor pain and prevent suffering. *Journal of Midwifery and Women's Health, 49*(6), 489–504.

Simkin, P., Bolding, A., Keppler, A., & Durham, J. (2010). *Pregnancy, childbirth, and the newborn: The complete guide* (4th ed.). Minnetonka, MN: Meadowbrook.

Simmons, S. W., Cyna, A. M., Dennis, A. T., & Hughes, D. (2007). Combined spinal-epidural versus epidural analgesia in labour. *Cochrane*

Database of Systematic Reviews, Issue 3. Art. No.: CD003401. doi:10.1002/14651858.CD003401.pub2.

Simpson, K. R., & Thorman, K. E. (2005). Obstetric "conveniences": Elective induction of labor, cesarean birth on demand, and other potentially unnecessary interventions. *The Journal of Perinatal and Neonatal Nursing*, *19*(2), 134–144.

Sjoblom, I., Nordstrom, B., & Edberg, A. (2006). A qualitative study of women's experiences of home birth in Sweden. *Midwifery, 22*(4), 348–355.

Slade, P., Macpherson, S. A., Hume, A., & Maresh, M. (1993). Expectations, experiences and satisfaction with labor. *British Journal of Clinical Psychology, 32*(4), 469–483.

Smyth, R. D., Alldred, S. K., & Markham, C. (2007). Amniotomy for shortening spontaneous labour. *Cochrane Database of Systematic Reviews*, Issue 4. Art. No.: CD006167. doi:10.1002/14651858. CD006167.pub2.

Soliday, E., McCluskey-Fawcett, K. A., & O'Brien, M. (1999). Postpartum affect in new mothers and fathers. *American Journal of Orthopsychiatry, 69*(1), 30–38.

Steer, P. J. (2008). Has electronic fetal heart monitoring made a difference? *Seminars in Fetal and Neonatal Medicine, 13*(1), 2–7.

Stewart, P., Kennedy, J. H., & Calder, A. A. (1982). Spontaneous labour: When should the membranes be ruptured? *BJOG: An International Journal of Obstetrics & Gynaecology, 89*(1), 39–43.

Stoll, B. J., Hansen, Fanaroff, A. A., Wright, L. L., Carlo, W. A., Ehrenkranz, R. A., Lemons, J. A. et al. (2002). Changes in pathogen causing early-onset sepsis in very low birth weight infants. *New England Journal of Medicine, 347*(4), 240–247.

Stolte, K. (1987). A comparison of women's expectations of labor with the actual event. *Birth, 14*(2), 99–103.

Strauss, A., & Corbin, J. (1990). *Basics of qualitative research: Grounded theory procedures and techniques*. Newbury Park, CA: Sage.

Su, M., McCleod, L., Ross, S., Willan, A., Hannah, W. J., Hutter, E. K. et al. (2007). Factors associated with maternal morbidity in the Term Breech Trial. *Journal of Obstetrics and Gynaecology Canada, 29*(4), 324–330.

Taffel, S. M., Placek, P. J., Moien, M., & Kosary, C. L. (1991). 1989 U. S. cesarean section rate steadies—VBAC rate rises to nearly one in five. *Birth, 18*(2), 73–77.

Towner, D., Castro, M. A., Eby-Wilkens, E., & Gilbert, W. M. (1999). Effect of mode of delivery in nulliparous women on neonatal intracranial injury. *New England Journal of Medicine, 341*(23), 1709–1714.

Tuffnell, D. (2010). Place of delivery and adverse outcomes. *British Medical Journal, 341*, c5560.

U.K. Home Birth Reference Site (2011). Home birth in the U.K. Retrieved from http://www.homebirth.org.uk/homebirthuk.htm.

United States Centers for Disease Control and Prevention [CDC]. (1999a). Ten great public health achievements—United States, 1900 to 1999. *Morbidity and Mortality Weekly Report, 48*, 241–243. Retrieved from http://www.cdc.gov/mmwr/preview/mmwrhtml/00056796.htm.

United States Centers for Disease Control and Prevention [CDC]. (1999b). Achievements in public health, 1900–1999: Healthier mothers and babies. *Morbidity and Mortality Weekly Report, 48*, 849–858. Retrieved from http://www.cdc.gov/mmwr/preview/mmwrhtml/mm4838a2.htm.

United States Centers for Disease Control and Prevention [CDC]. (2002). Prevention of perinatal group B streptococcal disease. *MMWR Morbidity and Mortality Weekly Report, 51*(RR 11), 1–22. Retrieved from http://www.cdc.gov/mmwr/preview/mmwrhtml/rr5111a1.htm.

United States Centers for Disease Control and Prevention & Health Resources and Services Administration. (2009). *Healthy People 2010, 16: Maternal, Infant, and Child Health.* Retrieved from http://www.scribd.com/doc/22593242/Healthy-People-2010-Maternal-Infant-and-Child-Health.

United States Department of Health and Human Services, Food and Drug Administration [FDA]. (1998, May 21). *FDA public health advisory: Need for caution when using vacuum assisted delivery devices.* Retrieved from http://www.fda.gov/MedicalDevices/Safety/AlertsandNotices/PublicHealthNotifications/UCM062295.

United States Food and Drug Administration [FDA]. (1981). Statement on use of pelvimetry X-ray examination. *FDA Drug Bulletin, 11*(3), 22.

United States National Center for Health Statistics. (1999). *Vital statistics of the United States, 1993. Vol. 1, Natality*. Retrieved from http://www.cdc.gov/nchs/data/vsus/nat93_1.pdf.

United States National Institute of Child Health and Human Development Research Planning Workshop. (1997). Electronic fetal heart rate monitoring: Research guidelines for interpretation. *American Journal of Obstetrics & Gynecology, 177*(6), 1385–1390.

United States National Institutes of Health [NIH]. (1981). Consensus development conference on cesarean childbirth, sponsored by the National Institute of Child Health and Development (1980, September). NIH Publication #82-2067. NIH: Bethesda, MD.

United States National Institutes of Health [NIH]. (2006). State-of-the-science conference statement on cesarean delivery on maternal request. *NIH Consensus Science Statements, 23*(1). Retrieved from http://consensus.nih.gov/2006/cesarean.htm.

United States National Institutes of Health [NIH]. (2010). Consensus development conference statement on vaginal birth after cesarean: New insights, final statement. Retrieved from http://consensus.nih.gov/2010/vbac.htm.

University of Washington, Anesthesiology & Pain Medicine. (2010). Epidural anesthesia: Technique. Retrieved from http://depts.washington.edu/anesth/education/resources/regional/epiduraltechtext2.html.

van Doesum, K. T., Riksen-Walraven, J., Hosman, C. M., & Hoefnagels, C. (2008). A randomized controlled trial of a home visiting intervention aimed at preventing relationship problems in depressed mothers and their infants. *Child Development, 79*(3), 547–561.

Ventura, S. J., Martin, J. A., Curtin, S. C., & Mathews, T. J. (1999). Births: Final Data for 1997. *National Vital Statistics Reports, 47*(18). Hyattsville, MD: National Center for Health Statistics. Retrieved from *www.cdc.gov/nchs/data/nvsr/nvsr47/nvs47_18.pdf.*

Veurink, M., & de Jong-van den Berg, L. T. (2005). The history of DES, lessons to be learned. *Pharmacy World Sciences, 27*(3), 139–143.

Villar, J., Valladares., E., Wojdyla., D. (2006). Caesarean delivery rates and pregnancy outcomes: The 2005 WHO global survey on maternal and perinatal health in Latin America. *Lancet, 367*(9525), 1819–1829.

Vincent, M. (2005). Amniotomy: To do or not to do? *Midwives: The Official Journal of the Royal College of Midwives, 8*(3), 228–229.

Waldenstrom, U. (2003). Women's memories of childbirth at two months and one year after the birth. *Birth, 30*(4), 248–254.

Wax, J. R., Pinette, M. G., & Cartin, A. (2010). Home versus hospital birth—Process and outcome. *Obstetrical & Gynecological Survey, 65*(2), 132–139.

Wei, S-Q., Luo, Z-C., Xu, H., & Fraser, W. D. (2009). The effect of early oxytocin augmentation in labor: A meta-analysis. *Obstetrics and Gynecology, 114*(3), 641–649.

Wei, S., Wo, B. L., Xu, H., Luo, Z. C., Roy, C., & Fraser, W. D. (2009). Early amniotomy and early oxytocin for prevention of, or therapy for, delay in first stage spontaneous labour compared with routine care. *Cochrane Database of Systematic Reviews*, Issue 2. Art. No.: CD006794. doi:10.1002/14651858.CD006794.pub2.

Wertz, R. W., & Wertz, D. C. (1989). *Lying in: A history of childbirth in America, expanded edition.* New Haven, CT: Yale University Press.

Wheeler, T. L., & Richter, H. (2007). Delivery method, anal sphincter tears, and fecal incontinence: New information on a persistent problem. *Current Opinion in Obstetrics and Gynecology, 19*(5), 474–479.

Wiegers T. A., van der Zee, J., & Keirse, M. J. (1998). Maternity care in the Netherlands: The changing home birth rate. *Birth, 25*(3), 190–197.

Williams, B. (1994). Patient satisfaction—A valid concept. *Social Science and Medicine, 38*(4), 509–516.

Williams, C., Sandall, J., Lewando-Hundt, G., Heyman, B., Spencer, K., & Grellier, R. (2005). Women as *moral pioneers*? Experiences of first trimester antenatal screening. *Social Science and Medicine, 61*(9), 1983–1992.

Wittmann-Price, R. A., & Bhattacharya, A. (2008). Reexploring the subconcepts of the Wittmann-Price Theory of Emancipated Decision Making in women's healthcare. *Advances in Nursing Science, 31*(3), 225–236.

Wong, C. A. (2009). Advances in labor analgesia. *International Journal of Women's Health, 1,* 139–154.

World Bank. (1993). *World development report 1993: Investing in health.* New York: World Bank and Oxford University Press. Retrieved from http://www-wds.worldbank.org/external/default/WDSContentServer/WDSP/IB/1993/06/01/000009265_3970716142319/Rendered/PDF/multi0page.pdf.

World Health Organization [WHO]. (1996). *Care in normal birth: A practical guide.* Retrieved from http://whqlibdoc.who.int/hq/1996/WHO_FRH_MSM_96.24.pdf.

World Health Organization [WHO]. (2005). The world health report 2005—Make every mother and child count. Retrieved from http://www.who.int/whr/2005/whr2005_en.pdf.

World Health Organization [WHO]. (2006a). *Integrated management of pregnancy and childbirth. Pregnancy, childbirth, postpartum and newborn care: A guide for essential practice* (2nd ed.). Geneva: WHO.

World Health Organization [WHO]. (2006b). *Neonatal and perinatal mortality: Country, regional, and global estimates*. Geneva: World Health Organization. Retrieved from http://www.who.int/making_pregnancy_safer/publications/neonatal.pdf.

World Health Organization & the Pan American Health Organization. (1985). Appropriate technology for birth. *Lancet, 2*(8452), 436–437.

Xu, J. Q., Kochanek, K. D., Murphy, S. L., & Tejada-Vera, B. (2010). Deaths: Final data for 2007. *National Vital Statistics Reports, 58*(19). Hyattsville, MD: National Center for Health Statistics. Retrieved from *www.cdc.gov/NCHS/data/nvsr/nvsr58/nvsr58_19.pdf.*

Yin, R. K. (2008). *Case study research: Design and methods* (4th ed.). Thousand Oaks, CA: Sage.

Zhang, J., Troendle, J., Mikolajczyk, R., Sundaram, R., Beaver, J., & Fraser, W. (2010). The natural history of the normal first stage of labor. *Obstetrics and Gynecology, 115*(4), 705–710.

Index